Spirituality, Suffering, and Illness

Ideas for Healing

LORRAINE M. WRIGHT, RN, PhD

Professor Emeritus of Nursing
University of Calgary

F. A. DAVIS COMPANY · Philadelphia

F. A. Davis Company
1915 Arch Street
Philadelphia, PA 19103
www.fadavis.com

Printed in Canada

Last digit indicates print number: 10 9 8 7 6 5 4 3 2 1

Production Editor: Jessica Howie Martin
Cover Designer: Joan Wendt
Publisher: Lisa B. Deitch
Developmental Editor: Diane Blodgett, Michelle L. Clarke

As new scientific information becomes available through basic and clinical research, recommended treatments and drug therapies undergo changes. The author and publisher have done everything possible to make this book accurate, up to date, and in accord with accepted standards at the time of publication. The author, editors, and publisher are not responsible for errors or omissions or for consequences from application of the book, and make no warranty, expressed or implied, in regard to the contents of the book. Any practice described in this book should be applied by the reader in accordance with professional standards of care used in regard to the unique circumstances that may apply in each situation. The reader is advised always to check product information (package inserts) for changes and new information regarding dose and contraindications before administering any drug. Caution is especially urged when using new or infrequently ordered drugs.

Library of Congress Cataloging-in-Publication Data

Wright, Lorraine M., 1944-
    Spirituality, suffering, and illness: ideas for healing/Lorraine M.
      Wright. p. ; cm.
    Includes bibliographical references and index.
    ISBN 0-8036-1171-4 (pbk. : alk. paper)
    1. Nurse and patient. 2. Suffering. 3. Spirituality. 4. Nursing.
5. Palliative treatment.
    [DNLM: 1. Pain—nursing. 2. Spirituality. 3. Stress, Psychological—
nursing. 4. Nurse-Patient Relations. 5. Nursing Care—methods. WY
87 W951s 2005] I. Title.
    RT86. 3.W756 2005
    610. 73' 06'99—dc22

                                  200401201

To the loving memory of my mother, Hazel Jean Schollar Wright, who has taught me more than any other person about suffering in the midst of serious illness. Despite her suffering, my mother's spirit still maintained a desire and joy for life and living. I miss her very, very much.

About the Author

LORRAINE M. WRIGHT, RN, PhD, is a Professor Emeritus of Nursing, University of Calgary, Calgary, Alberta, Canada. She is also an author, a consultant, and a marriage and family therapist. In 1982, she established the Family Nursing Unit within the Faculty of Nursing, University of Calgary, and she was the Director for 20 years. The Family Nursing Unit is a unique outpatient clinic for the treatment and study of families suffering with serious physical or mental illness.

Dr. Wright is the author of numerous articles and book chapters. She is also co-author of *Nurses and Families: A Guide to Family Assessment and Intervention* (4th ed, 2005) and *Beliefs: The Heart of Healing in Families and Illness* (1996), as well as co-editor of *The Cutting Edge of Family Nursing* (1990), *Families and Chronic Illness* (1987), *Families and Life-Threatening Illness* (1987), and *Families and Psychosocial Problems* (1987).

She serves on the Editorial Board of the *Journal of Family Nursing* and as Advisory Editor of the journals *Families, Systems and Health* and *Contemporary Family Therapy: An International Journal,* and she previously served on the Editorial Board of the *Journal of Marriage and Family Therapy*. Dr. Wright is a much sought-after speaker at family nursing, family therapy, and family health conferences and has given more than 300 presentations in Europe, Asia, Australia, Israel, and North America.

Dr. Wright is a member of the Canadian Nurses Association and the American Academy of Family Therapy and is an Approved Supervisor, Clinical Member, and Fellow of the American Association for Marriage and Family Therapy.

For more information about Dr Lorraine M. Wright's professional contributions, see the Websites: *www.familynursingresources.com* and *www.ucalgary.ca/nu/fnu*

E-mail: *lmwright@ucalgary.ea*

FOREWORD

This work takes the subject and experience of suffering and spirituality to a new level, penetrating the very lives of the author and those near and dear to Lorraine Wright as family, friends, acquaintances, and patients. She brings the Buddhist teaching and understanding that suffering transforms to life, bringing entirely new living, if not loving, insights into this ineffable human dilemma. Wright helps us to listen and hear more clearly the voices of those who suffer, revealing to us a "pedagogy of suffering" that we as health professionals and practitioners can learn perhaps only from those who are living in that space. These profound personal stories ground this work in such a way that we are invited into the "ultimate questions" without being overwhelmed, rather softened and humbled by their gift of grace. Wright's stories become our stories through the universality revealed by the individuality and the paradox of courage, grace, and healing as we experience joy and sorrow, enriching and alchemically altering human life and its mystery of being.

As Wright unfolds the mystery of suffering, she uncovers the unmistakable connection that suffering and spirit are one. She clarifies and integrates this insight and knowledge through her Trinity Model, revealing the inseparable relationship between suffering, spirit, and beliefs. The personal and professional poignancy of this work moves from testimony to message. The message in this work intersects with wisdom traditions, unending quests of perennial philosophy, and human questioning across time. These insights have a timeless, yet contemporary message of knowing that merges the paradox of opposites and unites spirit with joy and sorrow. The work illuminates the paradox of the human condition. Through her perennial wisdom and personal stories we find a work that comes alive with voices and the energy of love, hope, courage, joy; ultimately we understand the transformation of individual lives through living out their suffering and spirit. In the end, these stories and voices of transformation both inform and transform us all.

Jean Watson, RN, PhD, HNC, FAAN
Distinguished Professor of Nursing
Murchinson-Scoville Chair in Caring Science
University of Colorado Health Sciences Center
Denver, Colorado
Jean.watson@uchsc.edu

Acknowledgments

This is one of my favorite pages in the book. It is the page where I can step aside from the content for a moment and remember all who contributed so generously and thoughtfully to this project. Although the words on this page may be few, my appreciation, gratitude, and thankfulness are beyond words.

Special thanks and appreciation to:

The individuals and families in my professional practice with whom I have been privileged to assist and to learn from for more than 30 years. Their illness stories and their suffering have taught and changed me as a clinician, a nurse educator, and a woman. The collection of illness stories that I carry within me has profoundly softened my heart; touched my spirit; and, I believe, made me a better clinician, educator, and person. The clinical stories of families suffering with illness that I have retold in this book give the ideas their texture and richness. I am confident that the marvelous contribution of these individuals and families will inspire and ripple throughout many nurses' and other health-care professionals' practice.

Lisa B. Deitch, Publisher, Nursing Department, F. A. Davis Company, who competently watched over the project and is such an encouraging and personable publisher and person. Even her e-mails that said "Don't even THINK about going on the golf course" were just what I needed.

Diane Blodgett and Michelle L. Clarke, Developmental Editors, who never let me lose sight of those deadlines and were, as usual, very efficient in readying the manuscript for production.

Jessica Howie Martin, Production Editor, whose attention to detail was amazing.

Dr. Deborah McLeod, who generously contributed Chapter 3, "Spirituality and Illness in the Professional Literature," to make a most significant and comprehensive offering. In addition, I have included several of her understandings and reflections from her lovely piece of doctoral research.

Thelma Midori, Giezelle Pash, Barbara Pitcher, Suzanne Truba, Anne Marie Levac-Wolfert, Dr. Chintana Wacharasin, and Sheldon Walker, special friends and colleagues, and my amazing nephew, Ryan T. Wright, all of whom graciously and generously accepted my invitation to share their reflections and thoughts about suffering and spirituality within and outside the context of illness. Your contributions were poignant, reflective, and heartfelt. I learned from each of you, and I thank you.

Dr. Fabie Duhamel, Dr Maureen Leahey, and Joanne Stalinski, dear friends and colleagues. I offer my sincere thanks for your willingness to review and edit all of the chapters! Your thoughtful comments and conscientious critique have made this a much smoother, clearer, and, I hope, more useful book. I now look forward to

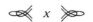 *x*

spending more time with each of you on the golf course if you are up to the challenge. I also wish to thank the two reviewers who accepted the invitation by F. A. Davis to critique my manuscript and, in so doing, have increased the clarity of ideas offered in this book.

Dr. Janice Bell, great friend and colleague, with whom I have shared a common mission to conserve and preserve family life in the midst of suffering from serious illness through many, many years of meaningful and rewarding work with graduate nursing students, and families in the Family Nursing Unit, University of Calgary, and also in our wonderful international teaching opportunities to health-care professionals. You have been such a strong supporter of my ideas and ambitions, whether overly small or overly grandiose. Dr. Nancy Moules, my newest colleague and friend in the Family Nursing Unit, who has brought her expertise about grief and grieving families. I appreciate your constant interest and passion for the work.

Graduate masters and doctoral nursing students in the Family Nursing Unit, who so willingly opened space to our nursing practice models and spiritual care practices. I am particularly grateful to Juliet Thornton, RN, MN, who was one of the clinicians for the families described in this text, and who gave so much of her knowledge, her compassion, and herself. I am also grateful to recent doctoral graduates, Dr. Deborah McLeod and Dr. Lori Limacher, whose beautiful pieces of research further contributed to the ideas offered in this text.

And finally, but essentially, friends Myrna Fraser and Marsha and Dr. Michael Laub, Dr. Wendy L. Watson and family members Marcy and Derek Borgford, Bob and Carol Wright, Erin and Doran Wright, and Dad and Marge Wright, who provided the personal support, interest, and caring that are so necessary to complete a book project. Each of you in your own way contributed to my ability to write this book!

Contributor

Deborah L. McLeod, RN, PhD
Clinician Scientist
QEII Health Sciences Centre
Cancer Care Program
Halifax, Nova Scotia, Canada

Reviewers

Brother Ignatius Perkins, OP, DNSc, MA ED, RN
Professor and Chair, School of Nursing
Dean, College of Health and Natural Sciences
Spalding University
Louisville, Kentucky

Cindy Parsons, MS, ARNP, BC
Adjunct Faculty
College of Nursing
University of South Florida College
Tampa, Florida

Contents

Introduction   *xvii*

1 Spirituality, Suffering, and
   Illness in Everyday Life   *1*

2 Reflections and Learning about
   Suffering   *35*

3 Spirituality and Illness in
   Professional Literature   *63*

4 The Trinity Model: Beliefs,
   Suffering, and Spirituality   *109*

5 Clinical Practices that Optimize
   Healing: Creating and Opening
   Space for Suffering and
   Spirituality in Conversations
   about Illness   *147*

6 Connecting the Personal and
   the Professional in Mattersof
   Suffering, Spirituality, and
   Illness   *193*

Epilogue   *213*

Index   *217*

Introduction

This is a book about spirituality, suffering, and illness. To help illustrate the connection between these three concepts, I chose the painting "The Doctor" by Sir Luke Fildes for the cover. I believe that it poignantly and persuasively invites us into the world of spirituality, suffering, and illness. Indeed, I think this powerful painting could be renamed "Suffering." The painting was inspired by the death of Fildes' eldest son, Phillip, who died Christmas morning, 1877. The painting has a happier ending than did real life, because the child in the painting has survived through the night and dawn is now breaking. Fildes made these comments about his painting: "At the cottage window the dawn begins to steal in—the dawn that is the critical time of all deadly illness—and with it the parents again take hope into their hearts, the mother hiding her face to escape giving vent to her emotion, the father laying his hand on the shoulder of his wife in encouragement of the first glimmerings of the joy which is to follow" (Wilson, 1997, p. 90).

To my knowledge, this is the first text for nurses and other health professionals that acknowledges the relationship between suffering and spirituality and provides a comprehensive discussion of the importance of these concepts within the context of illness. It also emphasizes the impact and influence of the family when serious illness arises rather than focusing on only the individual. The connection between suffering and spirituality is perhaps illuminated best through actual clinical examples of persons experiencing illness, which are sprinkled generously throughout this text.

Suffering and Spirituality in the Context of Illness

Nurses form relationships with individuals, families, and communities to promote health and alleviate or diminish suffering. Indeed, I believe that the very heart or essence of nursing is the encounter with suffering. Traditionally, nursing has professed to apply holistic approaches to caring for others and themselves and offering interventions that incorporate the biopsychosocial-spiritual domains of life. However, the spiritual domain has often been neglected, overlooked, or forgotten by nurses and other health professionals, even though spirituality has been found to play a key role in health and illness. Illness and suffering lead one into the spiritual domain of life.

In this text, the term "spirituality" designates the human desire for a sense of meaning, purpose, connection, and fulfillment through intimate relationships and life experiences. When serious illness arises in the life of an individual, it is usually accompanied by suffering. Frequently an experience of suffering leads one into the spiritual domain and invites questions about the big issues in life, such as: Why do I have this serious illness? How will my family cope? Why did my life have to change so abruptly? Why is this happening to me?

Nurses need to be prepared to respond with spiritual sensitivity to clients, family members, and communities who have or are experiencing serious illness, death, addiction, abuse, and environmental or terrorist catastrophes and to learn what kinds of spiritual conversations and practices can assist or inhibit healing.

This book provides a framework of knowledge, values, skills, and experiences for nurses seeking to connect suffering and spirituality. It explores and examines the role of spirituality in suffering and healing and vice versa. Readers are given an opportunity to participate in an open and critical reflection on the spiritual experiences of patients, caregivers, nurses, health professionals, and themselves. In addition, they are invited to reflect on their own spirituality and how it may affect their health care and relationships with others.

Some Background and Evolution of Thinking and Clinical Research

This book is the next logical progression in my theoretical, research, and clinical practice ideas for assisting individuals and families who are suf-

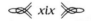

fering with serious illness. F. A. Davis Company has supported my ideas by publishing four editions of my co-authored book with Dr. Maureen Leahey entitled *Nurses and Families: A Guide to Family Assessment and Intervention,* with the most recent edition in 2005. In that text for general practice nurses working with families, we have a subcategory called "Religion and Spirituality" within the Calgary Family Assessment Model. The *Nurses and Families* text provides a brief description and definition of spirituality and religion and a few examples of questions that could be asked of a family. However, it is very limited in its discussion about this topic because that is not the focus of that particular text. However, one thing that *Nurses and Families* and this new text have in common is that they both are "how-to" books.

In 1996, Drs Wendy L. Watson, Janice M. Bell, and I co-authored a book entitled *Beliefs: The Heart of Healing in Families and Illness,* published by Basic Books, New York. From our clinical research, we became more convinced that what families believe about their illness is the most significant influence on how they cope with their illness. Therefore, in our *Beliefs* text, we dramatically expanded our ideas, knowledge, and understanding of beliefs. This learning was primarily gained through another research project that culminated in the writing of that text and in the development of the Illness Beliefs Model for advanced practice for health professionals. We encourage clinicians to explore a variety of beliefs about the illness experience. For example, we encourage the exploration of beliefs about etiology, prognosis, the role of family members and health professionals, and spirituality/religion. I mention my previous co-authored texts only because this new text flowed naturally from these two previous books.

Our *Beliefs* book was clearly focused on the beliefs of families and health-care professionals about illness. It was in this text that I began to write about the interconnection between beliefs, suffering, and spirituality. I emphasized the importance of health professionals exploring these domains when caring for persons with serious illness, but of course the primary focus of the book was on "beliefs."

For the past 10 years, I have been developing my own theoretical ideas, definitions, and descriptions of the concepts of suffering and spirituality. In my clinical practice and in the supervision of the practice of my graduate nursing students, I have been examining conversations of suffering and spirituality with persons experiencing serious illness. I have also been publishing and presenting these ideas about suffering and spirituality in the context of illness. More recently, I developed and taught a new course within the Faculty of Nursing, University of Calgary, called *Spirituality in Health and Illness.* In 2003, Dr. Deborah McLeod, one of our doctoral graduates in the Faculty of Nursing, University of Calgary, completed a very informative and helpful thesis entitled "Opening Space for the Spiritual: Therapeutic Conversations with Families Living with Serious Illness." She has generously contributed a chapter to this text, as well as some of her very useful ideas for nursing practice. Many aspects of my teaching, research, and practice have seemed to culminate in the writing of this new text.

Uniqueness of This Text

Other professional books have focused on *either* suffering *or* spirituality. The main distinguishing feature that differentiates this book from others is twofold. (1) This is the first textbook for nurses that connects suffering and spirituality concepts in a meaningful and thought-provoking manner. In some nursing texts on spirituality, the word *suffering* is not even listed in the index. (2) This text has very rich descriptions of actual clinical work with ideas for specific interventions that can be used to alleviate or diminish suffering within a spiritual domain. These descriptions of clinical work occurred with families in the Family Nursing Unit (*http:/:www.ucalgary.ca/nu/fnu*), a dynamic outpatient research and education clinic, Faculty of Nursing, University of Calgary. My colleagues, Dr. Janice Bell and Dr. Nancy Moules; my former colleague, Dr. Wendy Watson; and I have evolved a program of intervention research that has accompanied the clinical work with families experiencing serious illness. In addition, our doctoral students have contributed immeasurably to furthering our understanding by unpacking interventions that are used in the Family Nursing Unit.

A Tour of the Chapters

This book is conceptualized in three different phases. The first phase invites the reader to consider notions and experiences of spirituality and suffering in everyday life. In the second phase, the reader is gently brought from that reflection to one of being aware of the professional discussion of the concepts of suffering and spirituality within the context of illness. The third phase connects these two concepts and applies them in clinical practice through clinical examples, and offers clinical guideposts to help nurses bring forth conversations of suffering and spirituality that have a potential for healing.

Chapter 1 invites the reader to many reflections about what is considered suffering and spirituality in everyday life through various personal stories. These stories offer insights as to how suffering and spiritual beliefs and practices play out in interactions between ourselves and our families and friends.

Chapter 2 offers some highlights and learning from the professional literature and clinical experience about suffering and how it affects health and illness responses. This informs the reader of the current notions and broad range of opinions about what suffering is and a few thoughts about how to research suffering.

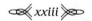

Chapter 3 presents a comprehensive review of the literature on spirituality and its relationship to health and illness. Useful distinctions are made between spirituality and religion. It also offers a caution to not objectify spirituality in nursing practice.

Chapter 4 offers a new model, namely, the Trinity Model, as a way of understanding the interconnectedness between beliefs, suffering, and spirituality. Two clinical examples are offered that beautifully illustrate this model and its trinity of concepts and how they may be observed and acknowledged in clinical practice.

Chapter 5 presents the clinical practices that embody a spiritual foundation necessary for reducing suffering from illness. The key ingredients for such practices include creating a healing environment; acknowledging that suffering exists; listening to, witnessing, and validating stories of suffering from illness; and, most important, creating a "reverencing" relationship between clinician and client. Several clinical vignettes are offered to illustrate of this type of practice.

Chapter 6 challenges nurses to connect their personal and professional lives in order to provide more genuine therapeutic conversations with their clients. Of course, the final chapter would not be complete without the final word, which is provided in the form of comments and statements from nurses, clients, and families about how their lives and relationships are changed when conversations about suffering and spirituality in the midst of serious illness are invited and connected.

My Hope for This Text

My sincere hope is that this book will provide nurses and other health-care providers with a thorough and comprehensive understanding of the interconnectedness of beliefs, suffering, and spirituality within an illness context. Therefore I offer a particular model, namely the Trinity Model (Chapter 4), to enable and encourage nurses to bring forth conversations about beliefs, suffering, and spirituality in clinical practice with ill persons and their family members. Knowing how to bring these conversations forth and what questions to ask can invite healing and diminish or alleviate emotional, physical, and spiritual suffering.

The influence of family members' spiritual and religious beliefs on their illness experiences has been one of the most neglected areas in health care despite the origins of nursing having a strong religious base. However, there is evidence that nurses are waking up to this neglected aspect in nursing practice. Increasing numbers of articles in professional journals and a handful of books with an emphasis on spirituality are now available. This book adds to that body of knowledge, but an important addition is the offering of very specific ideas of "how to" engage individuals and families in conversations about suffering and spirituality that have the potential to invite healing. It is my hope that this book can be a meaningful touchstone to provide the kind of compassionate care that nurses are so capable of providing and that clients and families are so eager to receive. In the end, both are blessed!

References

Wilson, S. (1997). *Tate Gallery: An Illustrated Companion.* London: Tate Gallery Publishing, p. 90.

Wright, L.M., & Leahey, M. (2005). 4th Ed. *Nurses and families: A guide to family assessment and intervention.* Philadelphia: F.A. Davis Co.

Wright, L.M., Watson, W.L., & Bell, J.M. (1996). *Beliefs: The heart of healing in families and illness.* New York: Basic Books.

1

Suffering, Spirituality, and Illness in Everyday Life

Only through experience of trial and suffering can the soul be strengthened, vision cleared, ambition inspired, and success achieved. The world is full of suffering, it is also full of overcoming it.

Helen Keller

Make everyday life your spiritual practice. When the milk boils over, when the bathroom flush doesn't work, when your colleague steals your idea and the lady standing next to you in the train is stepping on your toe, rejoice and give thanks!

Naomi Remen

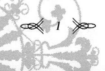

In this chapter, I invite the reader to reflect, ponder, and contemplate what constitutes suffering and spirituality in everyday life. It is in ordinary, everyday life that our encounters with suffering and spirituality often become extraordinary experiences. So, what does constitute and characterize suffering? What are our spiritual beliefs and practices? How might our spiritual beliefs and practices play out in our interactions with our families and friends? Are suffering and spirituality connected, and if so, how? How does one define suffering and spirituality? How is spirituality different from religion, or is it?

To understand the complexities and the many possible and varied answers to these questions, I have included some brief stories of suffering and spirituality in the everyday lives of a few friends and colleagues and of my nephew; all willingly and graciously contributed what they consider to be and have experienced as suffering and spirituality in their everyday lives. Of course, their stories are much more extensive and expansive than the few pages in this chapter permit, but the poignancy of their thoughts is profound, even if the accounts are short. Following their stories, ideas, beliefs, and ponderings, I add my own story for consideration.

These poignant stories and reflections of others, plus my own, compelled me to offer my definitions of suffering and spirituality in everyday life. Of course, with more experiences and more reflections, no doubt these definitions will change.

Definition of Suffering

My current definition of suffering is as follows: **physical, emotional, or spiritual anguish, pain, or distress. Experiences of suffering can include serious illness that alters one's life and relationships as one knew them; forced exclusion from everyday life; the strain of trying to endure; longing to love or be loved; acute or chronic pain; and conflict, anguish, or interference with love in relationships.**

Over the course of the last 5 years of my mother's life, when she suffered and endured her debilitating and limiting life experiences with multiple sclerosis, there were certain conversations we had that made such a profound impact on me that they have lingered long. One such conversation was on a day when I was wondering about the effect of my parents moving from their home in another city to the city where my brother, my sister-in-law, and I live. Our rationale was that, with our parents closer to us, we could be of more help and assistance. However, I worried if my mother were missing her home and friends in this other city. So one day I inquired, "Mom, do you miss Winnipeg?" And she responded with what became for me a great teaching moment: "No, Lorraine, I miss my life!"

Is it not the missing of a former life or the missing of what one had hoped for in life, with or without a serious illness, that is part of deep suffering? After periods of deep suffering, our lives as we knew them *are* changed forever!

Definition of Spirituality

My current definition of spirituality is **whatever or whoever gives ultimate meaning and purpose in one's life that invites particular ways of being in the world in relation to others, oneself, and the universe.**

I believe that everyone has some kind of spirituality or a particular way of being in the world. Some also embrace a religion. For the purpose of the discussion in this book, I have made a distinction between spirituality and religion, although for me, in my everyday life, they fit well being integrated. It is apparent in the stories that follow in this chapter that distinctions between and integration of religion and spirituality are clearly exemplified. Some of the storytellers readily identified their religion of Buddhism, Judaism, or Christianity and had integrated their spirituality and religion, whereas others made a distinction between their spirituality and religion. Others did not have the need to identify their religion, and some did not embrace any particular religion.

Definition of Religion

My current definition of religion is the **affiliation or membership in a particular faith community who share a set of beliefs, rituals, morals,** and sometimes a health code centered on a defined higher or transcendent power, most frequently referred to as God.

Religion, at its best, provides a home for the nourishment and development of a spiritual life. Most often this is the case, but sometimes it is not.

 Some clinical problems arise when religious stories, communities, and practices violate connectedness, hindering instead of helping a person to attain spirituality. (Griffith & Griffith, 2002, p. 18)

Religious beliefs and practices can be a source of great comfort to people who suffer from serious illness. However, it can also add to suffering if a person believes that his or her illness is a result of not having lived in congruence with his or her religious beliefs, or does not believe that his or her past deeds or behaviors are worthy of forgiveness or can be forgiven.

PERSONAL NARRATIVES OF SUFFERING AND SPIRITUALITY IN EVERYDAY LIFE

Through the following stories, it becomes readily apparent that suffering occurs both within and outside of the context of illness in as many and varied experiences as there are lives. It is also quite revealing that not all suffering in everyday life includes illness, nor does the experience of illness necessarily invite suffering. But when suffering does occur, it leaves a penetrating mark. And for all the people in these stories, their lives have profoundly changed as they have attempted to give meaning and understanding to these experiences. Spiritual thoughts, ponderings, wonderings, and changes in beliefs and behavior often followed closely behind their suffering, and in some instances even accompanied the suffering.

The first story is about a 50-year-old friend and colleague who recently experienced two acute illnesses that required surgery, but who states that these were not suffering experiences but rather "inconveniences" to her "exterior." She beautifully articulates that her suffering in everyday life was experienced when her "interior" was altered. She reflects first on observing the suffering of her family members, but realizes that her greatest suffering has been to have some of her religious beliefs challenged by a loved one.

There are many stories about suffering. I will share mine with you. My parents survived against all odds. Everyone else perished, not for anything they had done but only because they were Jews. My mother and father's Holocaust stories, tattooed on their hearts, bonded them in their suffering. There is much wisdom in the words of Nietzsche: "That which does not kill me makes me stronger." From my parents' suffering also came achievements that included their children, business, and friends. In this new country, their main goal was the well-being of their offspring. Even as a child, I always understood that their stories were pieces of my identity as well. As the years passed, our family grew alongside life's complexities. As in many families, health problems that accompany the aged and the not-so-aged struck us.

My mother did not suffer with her own three cancers as much as she suffered when her eldest daughter needed open-heart surgery or when chemotherapy took that same daughter's beautiful head of hair. During these times, my mother could not sing or dance when others could.

My 84-year-old father, once a businessman, fell into the grip of Alzheimer's 10 years ago. I wonder if he suffers. He seems to enjoy the simple things of life: eating his food; sitting in the yard; and attending family gatherings, where he repeats his repertoire of five questions that his family always politely answers as if it were the first time they had been asked.

In the past 5 years, I have experienced a laminectomy to remove a tumor in my spine and a parotidectomy to remove a tumor in my neck. Did I suffer? No, these inconveniences merely disrupted my exterior. My sense of self, that is, my interior, remained untouched. Perhaps my suffering has been watching my mother suffer when her children were ill, or was it observing the aging process slowly debilitate my parents? No, I do not suffer from these. My parents, despite their tragic family histories, did actualize their potential in life, and after all, is aging not a normal process?

But then one day some suffering caught me. A close loved one recently challenged my Judaism, my religious beliefs, and thus my interior. I had always believed that my parents' stories were not only a part of my identity but also a part of my loved ones' identity. I believed that their stories were our stories and that we are who we are because of them. Coming from a past where my grandparents, cousins, aunts, and uncles were robbed of their dignity, their lives, where they were just a number, where their histories did not matter, I vowed I would never again allow their history not to matter. Hence, this is now my greatest suffering, when my interior self was touched and challenged by the actions of a loved one who has chosen a different path that is not congruent with honoring our Jewish family heritage, especially regarding those who died in the Holocaust.

I had been taught that all people are responsible for each other. We create joy together. We cry together. Victor Frankl said, "Tears bear witness that a man had great courage, the courage to suffer." We suffer together and we hope together for world peace and for family harmony. That is what to me gives life its meaning and beauty.

In this heartfelt reflection of Jewish family history and suffering, this woman offers a beautiful insight that perhaps it is when our "interiors" suffer that we suffer the most. Some may even call this "interior" our spirit, our soul, or the very core of our being.

What is spirit? Spirit can be an enthusiasm and energy for living or someone's personality, attitude, or state of mind. It is also interpreted as a vital force that characterizes a living being as alive. It is a curious reflection that, on nursing notes in patient charts some years ago, it was common to read, "The patient is in good spirits." So even when illness is present, it does not always mean that one's spirit is dampened. But in this next story, another friend shares the thought that her experience of illness was indeed "soul searing and spirit killing."

I was seriously ill from 1995 to 1999. Due to an increasingly malignant [adrenal] Cushing's syndrome, my immune debility and hormonal holocaust manifested in a series of illnesses over a 2-year period: a ruptured spinal disc, diabetes, uncontrolled hypertension, disfiguring weight gain, muscular neuropathy, and osteoporosis. Following the adrenalectomy, I experienced surgically induced Addison's disease [which I still have], a fractured fibula, and thyroid cancer. I continue to monitor bone masses that were "discovered" on one of these diagnostic forays.

During this 2-year period, I had five lump scares. A rare benign adrenal lump caused the most systemic and enduring havoc. I argued to have a breast lump excised. Against great probability, a thyroid lump proved to be cancerous. And a benign bone lump grew and became two. My 4-year illness saga of "persistent adversity" (my physician's words) is the story before, during, among, and after these lumps.

The short answer to the question "What happened to my body?" is that I experienced multisystem failure.

The goofy answer is my body crapped out and I became a hormonal mistake. Perhaps my broken leg was a message to sit down to receive the news of thyroid cancer. It all fits.

The holistic answer is that the stress of work and a failing marriage brought my body to its knees. It yelled at me, "I can't do this any more."

Suffering had many faces when I was seriously ill:

Severe pain so sudden that I fell to the floor, drenched, unable to breathe, and thinking death was near

Not knowing, eternally waiting, longing for answers—even disastrous ones

Weakness, weariness, and hopelessness; the darkness of thinking "This is forever"

Darkness so complete that death would be a welcome light

When I had the energy and courage to persist with the question, "Why? Why is this happening to me?" my persistent illnesses and my suffering became my spiritual journey. And then I learned that joy and sorrow are one.

My suffering was a great source of learning, and the genesis of a new and ever-evolving view of who I am and why I am here. I am blessed with the ongoing questioning and answering.

At this moment, amazingly, I suffer no more. I consider myself cured, with some minor lifetime residual effects—glands that I had to give up and some muscle weakness to keep me active. (I do know that my life has been shortened, but only by a few days.) I cringe and ache for the suffering of others and sometimes despair for the world. But what, before my illnesses, I might have labeled "my suffering," I see in hindsight was only my anxiety, doubt, deep regret, disappointment, discouragement—but not the soul searing and spirit killing that I now know as suffering. In another lexicon, suffering is a shape-shifter!

Suffering has taken on a totally different meaning in the life of this friend's heart-wrenching illness story of "persistent adversity." She now discounts previous experiences that she thought of as suffering. And understandably so! This horrific illness story brought a deepening of the spirit to an already "deep soul."

But when illness has not been such a major "in-your-face" experience as it was for this woman, can we not still encounter suffering in everyday life? Here are the thoughts of another woman who does not cite illness as part of her life experiences with suffering, but nonetheless has experienced great anguish.

Suffering is significant to life. In my opinion, the law of the struggle is part of the master plan, part of the "set-up." I'll never quite understand why, but we learn so much about ourselves through our trials. I also know trials can make us into better people.

Being the owner of a small retail business and a single parent since my twins (boy and girl) were just 3 months old (now they are 29 years old and both married), periods of loneliness have been the great challenges in my life. Each has seemed unbearable at times, especially the role of sole provider for a family.

That which has strengthened me most is having faith in God and that He understands my weaknesses and hears my prayers. I fully believe that, inasmuch as I strive to make correct choices; do my best in my work, my family life, and help others; plus acknowledge God in all things, then that which comes into my life is for my highest good. But for me, the real challenge that comes from suffering is: do I press forward or give in to despair? To help bring me through these dark times, in addition to the much-needed and appreciated comfort of family and friends, is a scripture in the Old Testament in the Bible. It has given me great solace:

Trust in the Lord with all thine heart; and lean not unto thine own understanding. In all thy ways acknowledge him and he shall direct thy paths.

Proverbs 3:5, 6

It has been the daily challenges of being the sole wage earner as well as a single parent and the loneliness and angst that this can often bring that have invited suffering into my friend's life. It is obvious in her story that her great and admirable faith and spiritual beliefs have enabled her not to cave in to suffering even though she astutely and openly acknowledges that she does not fully understand why suffering is part of our human existence.

Great faith can also bring comfort and solace in times of tragic loss but is not necessarily accompanied by relief from grieving. Another friend faced this dilemma of faith and grief with the sad and premature loss of her husband. This dilemma requires and almost demands a mature heart and spirit, coupled with reflective thought, to open possibilities for healing. My friend possesses all of these. Read on.

My athletic, active, and always healthy husband of 25 years was diagnosed with colon cancer 1 month before Christmas. This brought initial surgery and then 5 years of religiously and courageously adhering to the prescribed treatment regimen, coupled with constant prayer by my husband and me, our family, and friends. But still he died at only 53 years old. I was his sole caregiver throughout his illness. The tragic and premature death of my spouse has caused me much suffering. But I have also come to understand suffering does not discriminate to only include death. As a parent, I found the greatest suffering comes when my children make choices that are not consistent with my values, teachings, and beliefs.

I have always had a strong belief in God and have found this to be a deeply meaningful relationship and comfort throughout my life. It was therefore instinctive for me to turn to this relationship for hope, direction, and perhaps some meaning to my "new life." Prayer and scripture study were familiar, comforting, and private. I have always viewed myself as fiercely independent and intellectually competent to deal with difficulties. My belief in God and my faith in His ongoing support were really not in question. What I found unfamiliar, however, was the intensity, frequency, and longevity of the grieving. The need to talk, and to have someone to listen, was also unfamiliar and left me feeling very vulnerable and needy.

My struggles and needs have been supported by what I call my "conversations of comfort." These are twofold. The first is my conversations with God through prayer. These conversations have changed as my struggles have intensified. They have become more frequent, more intense, more submissive, and more direct.

My other "conversations of comfort" are with people who invite conversation about my faith and beliefs about my suffering. These select and few people share my beliefs and provide safety for my questions, comfort to my pain, and redirection to my confusion.

My husband's physicians could not heal his body, but my conversations with others who allow me to speak of my suffering, my faith, and my belief in God are helping to heal my spirit. I believe that suffering not only allows us to grow, but draws us powerfully to our spiritual self. I have come to understand that, although suffering continues, peace can simultaneously be experienced as we explore and travel a spiritual journey to recovery.

The oddities and mysteries of life are played out in this next story of a somewhat younger friend. Although the previous friend shared her story of suffering and grieving the **loss** of life of her husband, the next friend provides a story of suffering about the inability, as yet, to **give** life and the questioning of whether this experience can be called "suffering." As you read her heartfelt words, you can again readily recognize and recall that these are descriptions of suffering, only dressed in different clothes. She recounts what some may call a "charmed life." However, when your heart's desire is to have your first child at the age of 41, all of the previous blessings of life lose their glitter.

In my life, I have been blessed with a supportive, spiritually strong family, close friends, good health, a rewarding career, and a steady, secure income. I have not personally encountered illness, divorce, poverty, chronic pain, or the death of a significant other. I have a wonderful husband whom I married just 2 1/2 years ago, who lavishes me with his good nature, his strong spirit, and his kind heart. In the scheme of things and all that life has and continues to bless me with, dare I use the word "suffer" at all in my life? Dare I use it to describe the last 2 years of unrelenting disappointment, helplessness, shame, inadequacy, and uncertainty associated with my infertility? Or could it be anything **but** suffering?

Five months into our marriage, I became pregnant and we were thrilled! It all happened perfectly as planned, and none too soon as I was 38 and my husband 37. Then, only 3 short months later, I miscarried. I was shocked. I was sad. I revisited every move I made or didn't make, searching for a cause. Uterine fibroids were the likely culprit and were promptly removed. I felt relief and anticipated another pregnancy and success soon. We tried "on our own" but still no success. We experimented with the least intrusive to the most intrusive of infertility treatments. Months were characterized by enormous hope and anticipated joy. (If I were pregnant, what would be the baby's birthday? How will we share the news with family and friends? Should I surprise my husband with the news by wrapping up the positive pregnancy test in a gold bracelet box?) Yet those very same months of anticipated joy were also met with repeated failure, unyielding disappointment, and a drained body and soul due to no successful pregnancy. Questions such as, "What's wrong with me?" "How much longer can we continue?" "Can it be that it is just not meant to be?" kept invading my mind.

On this emotional and physical roller-coaster ride, we asked ourselves lots of questions. Our doctor answered many of them. We now know how they measure follicles, count sperm, and grade eggs. We know about causes, chances, statistics, medications, hormone levels, and treatment options.

But the big questions, the searching questions, the searing questions, the ones that preoccupy me in the night, on the train ride to work, between intramuscular injections, blood work, and ultrasounds, are often less about causes and treatments. These questions are more about how to make meaning of and understand the reason for infertility in my life. My questions started with, "How could infertility strike ME, the second of five siblings with a father who places 14th in his siblings and a mother who places 4th in her family, which includes twins? My questions have now evolved to, "Is this going to be my cross to bear in life? What good will come of this? What does God want us to learn, to do, to give more of, to do less of? Does God have a different plan for us?"

> Throughout this process, we have prayed continually. In fact, in our short married life we have never prayed more together for anything. Our faith as a couple has been grounded through this process, and I often wonder if one purpose of our shared suffering has been a deepening of our faith. I do not believe that God's will is for us to suffer to become more spiritually connected, but indeed that has been one significant outcome. As we have become more open about our struggle, we've widened our prayer network. I have come to know who prays at work and who doesn't. I have had meaningful conversations with colleagues who I never knew believed so much in prayer, reassuring me that I was in theirs. We have been warmly comforted with the knowledge that prayers are said on our behalf from people we have yet to meet. My siblings tell me that we are in their prayers. There is no question in my mind that an outcome of our infertility has been a deepening of our faith and perhaps even the faith of others. Our faith has, over time, helped me to believe that we **will** make our family somehow, some way, some day. That hope gets me through my day-to-day "suffering."

For this close couple, the desire to bring life into the world through the bearing of children in a strong and loving marriage is a powerful and driving force; perhaps some may even say a spiritual force. The urgency to create a family is no doubt intensified because they have now both drifted into their 40s. I found that my friend's clear, disclosing, and open articulation of her evolving questions convinced me that suffering had definitely made its way into her husband's and her everyday life. When we suffer, we tend to have internal conversations with ourselves. But these conversations consist mostly of questions, not statements, about oneself, about the future, and about what life would mean and what it would be like without children, in the midst of keeping faith that this great miracle may still happen.

As my friends struggle and suffer with the disappointment of not yet **creating** life, my 30-year-old, single nephew celebrates the **keeping** of his life. However, this celebration and the great appreciation and meaning that he gives to his life were obtained only through intense suffering during the experience of a life-threatening illness.

The great Lance Armstrong wrote, "I want to die a hundred years old with an American flag on my back and the star of Texas on my helmet, after screaming down an alpine descent on a bicycle at 75 miles an hour" (Armstrong & Jenkins, 2000). I believe there are moments in everyone's life when they feel similar sentiments. I just so happened to feel this way very early in my life.

To understand my comments, I should give you some background. At the age of 2 or 3, I was diagnosed with aortic stenosis, a chronic condition that, for the most part, had very little effect on my life. In fact, I thought I was quite typical. As a true-blooded Canadian, I played hockey from a very early age until my teens. I participated in anything and everything that was physical.

I continued feeling "normal" until a little after my 15th birthday. At this point, I was having slight symptoms of a heart condition, and I was told I had to undergo open-heart surgery to widen one of my heart valves. I was more worried about the grotesque scar that the surgery would leave than the procedure itself. This is a characteristic teenage response to life-threatening surgery, I'm sure. Again, this all felt typical to me, and I absorbed this circumstance as if I was going off to a Disneyland. I told myself, "My friends aren't going to be there, but this should be cool." Life was back to normal within a few weeks after this surgery!

This all changed on May 12, 1996. I was a 23-year-old pseudo-student returning to university for the third time, taking my fourth major. Believe me, for a 23-year-old, this seems very emblematic. On that memorable day, I was visiting the student health center at the university for what I thought was the flu. Within 4 hours, I found myself admitted to the local hospital with bacterial meningitis. I realize the seriousness of the condition now, but at that time, I initially thought it was fairly typical or common. This abruptly changed after the doctors pinpointed exactly what was wrong with me.

I had contracted bacterial meningitis with the primary infection in my heart. I was told that this is atypical for the disease and, in fact, that it was life threatening! I knew this must be so because of how my family was reacting. My family is full of health-care professionals. They were showing signs of knowing the severity of my condition: they called frequently; my parents rushed to be with me; and I was told that many were praying for me.

I suppose this is when the self-reflection and self-doubt began. As my surgery was only 2 days away, I was lucky not to be tormented for too long, although I did not sleep at all. I was scared, very scared! I understand it is normal at this juncture to start thinking of spirituality and spiritual beliefs. I did not want to die at 23. I wanted to die at 100, playing hockey with the Canadian maple leaf on my chest.

At 6:30 AM on May 14, 1999, I underwent emergency open-heart surgery to repair the damage done by the disease. I awoke later in intensive care, suffering a great deal. Apparently, at some point after the surgery, one of my lungs had collapsed. I experienced extreme and excruciating pain that I cannot explain in words. Unfortunately, the pain medication did very little to help. It was my mother's touch that soothed me the most. Touch, I learned, is the best pain medication. It was my mother's gentle rubbing of my arm, holding my hand, and hearing her soft voice that helped me manage the pain. It is amazing how the energy and spirit of a person can truly be transformed to healing energy.

The idea of healing energy was solidified in my mind after the experience with my mother and the experience I had with an intensive care nurse. Because I was having problems breathing, they re-intubated me. After this procedure, my movements were very limited. This leaves one feeling not only in pain but extremely vulnerable. I'm sure this nurse understood this very well because every time that she came near my bed, she immediately held my hand. In fact, while in the room, she was rarely not in physical contact with me. This truly made the pain subside.

Since this hospital experience, I have reflected a great deal on how this experience has changed my life and my beliefs. I believe it made three significant impacts on my life. First, I believe that the daily decisions I make affect not only myself but also those I love. Second, I have a strong belief that things happen for a reason, even open-heart surgery. Finally, I have a fervent belief in the power of the healing touch. I realize that these may not be unique beliefs, but they were not part of my beliefs before my life-threatening illness. One last footnote: this 23-year-old college dropout has parleyed his new beliefs and priorities into obtaining an MBA and teaching college at the University of Montana, where my life-threatening crisis happened 7 years ago. Even a PhD might be in my future. Who would've figured?

Of course, I am thrilled and deeply grateful that my nephew's life was spared. I am also in admiration of the meaning he found in the suffering from his life-threatening illness experiences that have benefited his life in such a positive way.

The next reflection is a lovely way to conclude these stories and reflections of suffering from others. This friend offers her ideas and beliefs about suffering and spirituality that are very influenced by and grounded in her Buddhist beliefs.

I live in Thailand, and I was raised in a Buddhist family and internalized Buddhist beliefs into my life. I am very proud of being born in a supportive, good-spirited, and good-natured family. We have very strong family ties. My parents tried to teach their six children to control suffering by raising us to have a strong will and spirit and the necessary coping skills for suffering.

Our Buddhist beliefs teach us that our lives follow the path of Karma, which means that good Karma happens when we do good behaviors and thinking for others and ourselves and consequently create a life of happiness. In contrast, bad Karma occurs when we do unacceptable or inappropriate behaviors that bring about a bad life and suffering. Consequently, we try very hard not to hurt or to cause harm to others. Buddhism encourages us to be a good person and to make merit (doing good for others) in order to have a better life. Moreover, Buddhism invites people to practice neutrality by taking the middle road and not being extreme in thinking or behavior. We also try to accept others' beliefs and ideas for living.

Sometimes when I am suffering, I consider the bad Karma (things I did in the past in my life) that may be causing my suffering. In so doing, it helps me accept the suffering more easily and then live my life with less suffering.

Buddhism also teaches us how to cope with suffering by following four steps: (1) identify suffering, (2) consider possible causes of suffering, (3) find the appropriate way to reduce suffering, and (4) implement some solutions to release the suffering.

Some 15 years ago I underwent laminectomy due to a neurofibroma of my fourth cervical disc. From that treatment I should have experienced extreme suffering in my life, but I did not because, I believe, I had wonderful support from my family and friends as well as colleagues. In fact, it turned out that this critical time was an excellent chance for a reunion with my family and friends. In addition, I had faith and confidence that my good Karma would help me get through.

In everyday life as a single Thai woman with simplicity in my life, I am secure in my career and relationship with my family, close friends, and colleagues. I feel a low level of suffering when I am missing my loved ones, something is bothering me, or I am unable to finish a project at my work on time or complete something that is less than the expectations of myself or others.

In my opinion, suffering in human life could be rated from none at all to extreme suffering. It is a very subjective concept and depends on one's life experience, psychological structure, protective contexts (support systems and community), and one's religious and spiritual beliefs. My belief is that the way to cope with suffering relates and is connected to spirituality.

This lovely reflection from a Buddhist woman offers us the notion that we are not always subject to suffering from things that happen outside our control, but that there are times when we may invite our own suffering through the manner in which we live our lives. She also shares her experience with a potentially serious illness that was corrected by surgery, and how her own suffering was decreased and diminished by the presence and social support of family and friends.

I was incredibly moved by, and stand in deep awe and respect for, each of these powerful stories. One of the surprising experiences for me is that, although I am familiar with all of these stories, to read them on paper gave them a new light and a new understanding for me about suffering and spirituality. Some of my friends and family members have reported that the writing of their brief suffering narrative also gave them a new vision and meaning.

I would now like to add to these beautiful stories my story of how I have experienced suffering and spirituality in my everyday life.

I first experienced suffering from illness in my childhood. My English maternal grandmother, who lived with us, suffered chronic pain from rheumatoid arthritis. She had tremendous status and respect in our family by filling the role of "mother" by day while my mother worked outside the home with my father in our family business.

I observed the demoralizing suffering that one can experience from chronic pain, whether it is firsthand, as my grandmother suffered, or secondhand, as I emotionally suffered with her. I also learned that chronic pain controlled all of our lives, especially how well my brother and I would behave on any given day, how much my grandmother was able to "mother," and how we children were invited to be more compassionate because of having a pain sufferer in the family. My grandmother was the center of our family, but the chronic pain she suffered ruled even her. The disease severely disfigured her hands, caused her knees to be swollen much of the time, resulted in her walking with a limp, and dictated how well she was able to live her life on any given day. But those disfigured hands made us apple pie, weeded our garden, and lifted numerous cups of tea while we exchanged stories of our lives and relationships with her. However, I do not recall as a child hearing **her** stories of suffering with chronic pain. Perhaps I did not listen. Perhaps these stories were not told.

Now, however, I have several questions that I would eagerly ask of her. What meaning did she give to this life of chronic pain? What did she believe was the best treatment or healing for her pain? What did she believe helped to alleviate or diminish some of her suffering? What made it worse? What made it better? What help or hindrance was her spiritual and religious beliefs? Did she pray about her pain? What did she believe we grandchildren did to help or hinder her pain? Which was worse: emotional, physical, or spiritual pain? And what did she believe healthcare professionals did to help or hinder her pain? I wonder if conversations that may have included the answers to these questions would have contributed to some healing for both my grandmother and me.

Although there have been other illness experiences

and deaths over the years with friends, friends' parents, and, tragically, even children, the most profound shaping experiences of suffering was the 5-year ordeal of my mother's life as she, my father, other members of my family, and I dealt with the suffering and adversity of a cruel illness called multiple sclerosis. As my mother suffered, we as a family suffered with her. Initially, she suffered the most emotionally and spiritually in her wonderment. Why had this happened to her? What caused it? Later, it was her physical suffering that took prominence while emotionally and spiritually she became stronger. Even in her final year, when she was a quadriplegic, she never lost hope or faith that perhaps one day she would walk again. Her tenacious and determined spirit lifted my spirits, initially.

I observed and was amazed how my mother coped with this adversity with such courage, patience, and graciousness and an incredible noncomplaining attitude. She had the capacity, even amid a horrible, debilitating illness and chronic pain, to experience joy from small pleasures such as watching the birds through her window or enjoying *Wheel of Fortune* on television with my father. Here was a vibrant and enthusiastic woman who had worked until she was 72 years old, now confined to one room.

She constantly expressed her appreciation and gratitude for all that was done to care for her. I learned from my mother that suffering had the potential to refine and enable other qualities of her character to shine through. We were frequently amazed as a family how on many days, even when she could no

longer walk or feed herself, when we asked, "How
are you doing?" she would respond, "I have had a
wonderful day."

A wonderful day? How could she have a wonderful
day when she was not able to get out of bed on her
own, brush her hair, walk, feed herself, or even
scratch her nose? I needed to understand more, so
one day I asked her, "Mom, what keeps you going?"
She said, "The love of my family, especially your father. He is so good to me! I just hope that I will not
become too much of a burden for my family or that
they will tire of visiting me." As I read my journal entries recounting my mother's words, I continue to be
amazed and in awe as I realize the power of love—
when illness robs you of all of your faculties and dignity, love sustains your spirit.

My own suffering over those 5 years took many
forms: sadness, anger, anxiety, and even moments of
great peace. There were many exacerbations with my
mother's illness, with each one leaving her more dis-
abled than before.

Just 1 year into my mother's ordeal, I wrote an e-
mail to a close friend and entitled it "DAMN MS." I
wrote, "Just got off the phone from my parents, and
yes, my mother IS having another MS attack. They are
going to try and avoid another hospitalization and
give her steroids on an outpatient basis, but it will depend on how the next few days go…her legs are
numb tonight and the pain is terrible. I must say that
my spirits have been knocked, my Dad sounded
knocked also. My poor Mom! What a damn illness! Is
this what it's going to be like from now on…?? I
sensed that my Mom is trying to be brave; my Dad

sounds defeated. Well, I think I'll make some mint tea and try and soothe my spirits. Keep my parents in your prayers and me too, OK?"

I am impressed and struck by my use of the word "spirit" to describe the effect of my suffering. Spirit and suffering were now connected in my personal life as well as my professional life.

And there were numerous such e-mails and entries in my journal over those 5 years! Thinking back about my own suffering that arose through the observing and witnessing of my mother's debilitation, pain, and suffering, plus witnessing the suffering of my father, there were particular markers that indicated my mother's life as she had known it was irreversible, and these markers deepened my suffering.

One such marker was a simple but powerful one indicating the changing of my mother's ability and participation in the world. It was the time that I bought her first dress with Velcro strips. My mother, with her magnificent and plentiful wardrobe, and as many shoes as Imelda Marcos, was now in clothes fastened with Velcro! I cried as I walked to my car following the purchase of her new dress with Velcro strips.

Another major marker for me was the day when my mother did not desire food or to eat any more. I knew this meant the end of her life was near. For this reason, I needed her to eat. But soon we discovered that she loved the nutrient drink Boost, and for a time that lifted my spirits because it seemed to keep death from the door. I would tease her that we would have to send her to Boost Anonymous because she was addicted to that drink. On the day before my mother passed away, her marvelous caregiver was feeding her

Smarties (M&M's) for breakfast. Smarties for breakfast! I was as happy and delighted to witness this unusual event as if she were enjoying a five-course meal.

Perhaps one of the most painful markers was the day when I prayed that my mother would be released from her body, if that were God's will. I could not believe that I could utter such a prayer. I had listened to family members of clients over the years relate their pleadings in similar kinds of prayers. But I could never, ever imagine having such a desire or prayer. But now here I was, wishing, thinking, and praying for the same thing. Whose suffering was I praying to release, my mother's or my own? In the final few days of my mother's life, watching her struggling to breathe in her tiny, emaciated body made me wish and pray for her death. And just a few days after this prayer, she did pass away. Were my prayers answered or was it simply "her time," the failing of her body, or all of these? I do not know, and it does not matter now.

As my sister-in-law hugged my father and me at my mother's bedside at the time of her death, she uttered these comforting words: "Free at last." Yes, my mother and all my family members were now indeed free at last. Free of the unrelenting suffering of those 5 years, but of course not free of the grieving that would begin. However, in the months and already some 4 years since my mother's death, I was and am amazed and surprised to learn, for me at least, that grieving is sweet compared with those years of suffering. And I have her sweet memories, sweet pictures, and my own sweet and private moments that I spend at my mother's graveside.

Concluding Thoughts

From these very compelling and heartfelt stories, it seems clear that suffering is life wrenching and life altering, yet it can even be life giving. Several of the contributors offer the notion that suffering often leads one on a spiritual journey or a turning toward spirituality and/or spiritual beliefs in a quest for meaning. In this quest, some discovered that suffering and joy are inextricably connected and even, surprisingly, on the same side of the coin.

 Even the most physical suffering is not strictly physical at all. It does not end in the physical realm where it began. It soaks into the heart and spreads. Suffering is finely connected to the versatile and permanent self, the spirit. Suffering is a spiritual matter. (Brickey, 2001, p. 47)

The idea that suffering becomes a spiritual matter was a significant component of all of the stories offered in this chapter, whether written by those who identify with particular religious faiths and traditions or by those not associated with any particular religious tradition. But all experienced a turning toward their own spirituality and spiritual beliefs. Yes, suffering does become a spiritual matter.

One recurring theme that I read in the suffering stories of friends, family, and myself is that, after the experiences of suffering, there are emotional, physical, and/or spiritual changes. No one is the same after experiencing deep suffering.

Perhaps this is because suffering does not seem to come with an easy road map for finding our way to understanding its existence or why we suffer at all in life's journey. There are no apparent signposts, no familiar terrain, and no detours. Even without a road map, perhaps one of the gifts of suffering is that it brings with it a particular depth and richness of thought. As one woman said, "I don't miss my suffering, but I do miss the quality of thought. I was more removed from the world and its trivia." Yes, suffering does invite a particular depth of thought, a particular sobering and humbling opportunity for growth, for change, and for a possible openness or invitation to spirituality.

As one of the contributors so poignantly said, "Suffering has many faces." No one person's suffering is the same as another's, nor do we arrive at the same meaning derived from suffering experiences. Even within similar cultures and similar religious traditions, the meaning that each person derives from his or her suffering is not necessarily the same. But suffering does seem to have a constant companionship with spirituality.

What is the message to take away from all of these powerful narratives? The first is the appreciation that suffering and spirituality are intricately connected. Another, I believe, is the need to develop our own spirituality and to realize that it has the potential to assist us enormously when suffering arises, particularly later in life, when illness and loss tend to occur with greater frequency and regularity. And in our professional practice, we need to remember that "meaning-centered" conversations with health professionals provide a critical boost to individuals and families to cope and manage serious illness. It is even more important for those nearing the end of their lives (McLain, Rosenfeld, & Breitbart, 2003). In my clinical practice with clients and their families, young and old, and even persons with just a few weeks or months to live, I have found that they can benefit from finding meaning and value in their lives through therapeutic conversations with health professionals that reduce or diminish suffering. It is never too late.

Thus, it is our great privilege as health professionals to assist those suffering—emotionally, physically, and spiritually—with serious illness, loss, and grief to find meaning, purposefulness, intimacy, and connections in their new and altered "everyday lives." I offer this chapter and these stories as a way of inviting you, the reader, to a more personal reflection on your own suffering and spirituality in everyday life. Your reflections will, I believe, open your mind, heart, and spirit to the ideas offered in this book; to the Trinity Model; and to the examples of families with whom I have worked in my professional practice that are presented in the chapters that follow. By the conclusion of this book, particularly in Chapter 6, it will become apparent that, in matters of suffering and spirituality, we cannot help but connect the personal and the professional.

References

Armstrong, L., & Jenkins, S. (2000). *It's not about the bike: My journey back to life.* New York: Putnam Publishing Group.

Brickey, W.E. (2001). *Making sense of suffering.* Salt Lake City: Deseret Books.

Frankl, V.E. (1962). *Man's search for meaning* (I. Lasch, Trans.). Boston: Beacon.

Griffith, J.L., & Griffith, M.E. (2002). *Encountering the sacred in psychotherapy: How to talk with people about their spiritual lives.* New York: The Guilford Press.

McLain, C.S., Rosenfeld, B., & Breitbart, W. (May 10, 2003). Effect of spiritual well-being on end-of-life despair in terminally-ill cancer patients. *The Lancet, 361*(9369).

2

Reflections and Learning about Suffering

Suffering completely fills the human soul and conscious mind, no matter if the suffering is great or little.

Victor Frankl

Suffering Is the Heart of Nursing

I submit that reducing or diminishing suffering is the center, the essence, and the heart of nurses' clinical practice and indeed a major part of all health professionals' practice. Therefore the ethical and obligatory goal of nursing must be to reduce, diminish, or alleviate (and, we hope, heal) emotional, physical, and/or spiritual suffering of patients and their family members. I believe that alleviation of suffering has always been the heart of nursing, but it has not always been recognized as such. Reed (2003), perplexed by the lack of attention to suffering by health-care professionals, offers the following poignant comment:

 How strange it seems that suffering and its relief, which are central to the mission of health care, are mentioned so infrequently in many hospitals and within the health-care delivery system. Although there is much talk in clinical conferences about treatment strategies, physical symptom management, and patient care outcomes, it would be quite remarkable to discover a case conference planned to address, "The Suffering of John T, Room 310." The successes of modern science convey the impression that suffering has been conquered, but sensitive observation in any health-care environment demonstrates that suffering is pervasively present. (Reed, 2003, p. 4)

Conversations about suffering are not routinely brought forth in nurses' encounters with families experiencing serious illness. To understand what prevents or impedes nurses from engaging their patients in conversations about suffering, a reflection by myself and an examination of what exists in the professional literature about suffering provide some clues.

Suffering is raw, personal, and deep. Suffering is not partial to any particular gender, race, or religion; it spares no one and favors no one. Suffering is seen in the young as well as the old. And suffering has a very demanding dimension. It continually begs for explanation about why it has occurred and how it can be endured. Suffering can mean to experience, undergo, or tolerate anguish, grief, loss, and/or unwanted or unanticipated change. The type of suffering within the context of illness needs to be told and talked about. However, too often patients and family members are encouraged to tell only their medical story or narrative. The *medical narrative* means to discuss the disease or condition, complete with medication, dosages, and tests, whereas the *illness narrative* is the story of suffering and the effects of this suffering on the individual, his or her relationships, and his or her world.

The capacity of health professionals to witness the stories of suffering in families is central to providing care; it is frequently the genesis of healing, if not curing (Frank, 1994; Kleinman, 1988). In working with individuals and families, nurses have an important opportunity to invite and witness stories within which a "domain of spirituality is encountered. This journey into spirituality manifests itself in the offering of reverencing, compassion, and love between and among family members and therapists" (Wright, 1999, p. 75). In the inviting and witnessing of stories, the spirituality that is embedded in our lived experience of the world addresses both nurses and patients' families.

The Emergence of Suffering in Illness

Serious illness is a wake-up call about life. It comes in many forms, such as chronic illness, life-threatening illness, and mental illness. It arouses the need to be known, to be heard, and to be validated—the need to know that one's life matters in the life of someone else and that the life one is living and has lived is worthwhile (Frank, 1994). These needs fuel the telling of individual and family members' experiences with illness. And these *illness experiences* have become known as *illness stories* or *narratives* (Kleinman, 1988).

It is within these illness stories that suffering looms. Nurses are always in the midst of a person's encounter with illness. They have the privileged opportunity to bring forth illness narratives in their conversations with persons suffering with illness. Questions like the following are essential to understand the effect, impact, and changes caused by illness in a person's life and relationships: "What changes, if any, have there been in your life since you were diagnosed with your serious illness? What has been the effect of this illness on your marriage and your family?" These types of questions address the suffering that is being endured and the systemic effects of that suffering. Sometimes questions can be made even more specific about suffering by simply asking, "Who in the family is suffering the most?" The responses to these types of questions quickly confirm that suffering IS the illness experience. Unfortunately, these types of questions are not part of most nurses' conversations with patients.

Suffering and Research

Frank (1994) suggests that the primary lesson the ill have to offer is the "pedagogy of suffering." These teachings compel us to offer healing nursing practices that relieve suffering. In addition, we are compelled to conduct research to further our knowledge about which nursing practices actually do diminish or relieve suffering.

To conduct research about suffering, we must first acknowledge the dramatic difference in daily living between nurses and those in their care. The seriously ill and their family members live in a world that is profoundly dissident from that of nurses. The ill and their family members experience a world where suffering becomes a constant companion, and frequently a tormenting and agonizing companion. This suffering manifests itself in many ways. For example, strained

family relationships, forced exclusion from everyday life, and the loss of one's former life become commonplace.

The alleviation of suffering has always been
the cornerstone of caring. Suffering gives "caring
its own character and identity, and all forms of
caring aim, in one way or another, to alleviate
suffering" (Lindholm & Eriksson, 1993, p.
1354). But what IS the best way to care for those
who are suffering? What do the seriously ill and
their family members convey about their suffering in conversations with health professionals?
Listen to the story of the suffering of a woman in
her late 40s who is experiencing the serious illness amyotrophic lateral sclerosis.

 I have suffered so many losses. In the 8 months
since my diagnosis, my legs and left hand and
arm are paralyzed and my right hand is deteriorat-
ing. My capability of speech is gone and I am having trouble swallowing. I depend on everyone to
do almost everything for me. But this is just the
summary of the physical list. What I have really
lost is *me*! It is like everything I love is being
moved out of my reach. Yet, I am still here in the
presence of my life, but unable to participate.

However, suffering does not occur in a vacuum
or in isolation. Suffering is linked to and intertwined with the beliefs that one holds about his
or her illness (Wright, Watson, & Bell, 1996). A
belief is the "truth" of a subjective reality that influences biopsychosocial-spiritual structure and
functioning (Wright et al., 1996). Individual beliefs of patients and family members are in-

volved both in the experience of suffering and in making inferences from suffering. Certain beliefs may conserve or maintain an illness; others may exacerbate symptoms; others alleviate or diminish suffering (Wright et al., 1996). For example, what family members and nurses believe about the patient's prognosis, diagnosis, or treatment and healing can enhance or diminish suffering.

But, again, what ideas and definitions are offered about suffering in the professional literature? Morse and Johnson (1991) offer the idea that suffering is a comprehensive concept that includes the experience of both acute and chronic pain, the strain of trying to endure, the alienation of forced exclusion from everyday life, the shock of institutionalization, and the uncertainty of anticipating the ramifications of illness. Other descriptions of suffering include despair, lack of strength, longing for home, longing for love, something that hurts, and breakdown of relationships.

Reed (2003), who offers another thoughtful description and definition of suffering, suggests that suffering is characterized by its symptoms and underlying substance. She therefore offers the definition of:

 ... suffering as a syndrome of some duration, unique to the individual, involving a perceived relentless threat to one or more essential human values creating certain initially ominous beliefs and a range of related feelings. (p. 11)

Suffering, Reed contends, is the matrix in which fears, altered beliefs, and related emotions develop and in which they are embedded. She also names four useful distinctions about the intensity of suffering: distress, misery, anguish, and agony. To my knowledge, Reed (2003) also offers the first proposed Model of Suffering in the literature.

One special friend and colleague, Sheldon Walker, on listening to my tales of writing this book, spontaneously sent me his creative and thoughtful definition of suffering. I believe he captures the "ordinary" of suffering as opposed to the often emotionally distant and removed professional definitions of suffering, although professional definitions are important to form a common language and a base for understanding among health professionals.

S U F F E R

S is for Sorrow. Sorrow is different from sadness. Sad people can be cheered up, distracted, told a joke, or soothed. When one feels sorrow, one is inconsolable. There is a kind of heaviness, or pain or disappointment that permeates one's very being. Its depth may lessen in intensity over time, but it never really leaves. Sorrow usually includes a sense of regret, a kind of self-recrimination over not having the power to prevent some disaster or loss. The idea persists that one should have the power to prevent some disaster or loss; the idea that one should have done something leaves a residue or regret.

U is for Unfair. One asks: "What combination of divine, or cosmic, or random forces led me to this sorry state? How is it that others escape pain or hardship, yet I am destined to endure disaster? Why me? Why do I deserve this? It does not seem fair."

F is for Fretting. Fretting is worrying about the catastrophe that has happened or is about to take place. Fretting keeps one awake at night and on edge during the day. To fret is to have hundreds of tiny pins pricking one's sense of peace.

F is for Fear. Fear believes that bad things do not happen just once. Bad things get worse. Circumstances will never be good again. "There are things that will hurt me. The world is not a safe place."

E is for Emptiness. Emotional emptiness is what happens when one cannot take anymore. It is a kind of resignation to floating on the battering currents of a stormy sea. One can flail no more. There is nothing left. There is a hole where joy once reigned.

R is for Ruminating. Ruminating is like that song or piece of music you cannot get out of your mind. The tape plays again and again. Ruminating and replaying unfortunate events tend to arouse the bodily reactions associated with fear, flight, or fight. A person cannot be calm and ruminating at the same time. Psychological and physiological functions are busy. There is no way to feel calm when repetitive thoughts are working away.

This is my acronym for what suffering entails.

Health professionals may deny patients' suffering because increasing numbers of persons define themselves as victims and as sufferers. Their wish for attention, resources, and compassion for situations that were once thought of as the vicissitudes of life or a consequence of one's own behavior may now impede nurses and other professionals from "suffering with" or showing compassion to sufferers. Individual beliefs of health professionals, patients, and family members are involved both in the experience of suffering and in making inferences of suffering.

In an eloquent and illuminating explanation of illness experiences, Frank (1995) offers another idea of how persons make meaning of their suffering. He asserts that people tell stories of their illness to make sense of their suffering and that when they turn their diseases into stories, they find healing.

From my clinical practice and research with families, I have come to strongly believe that talking about experiences with chronic pain can often alleviate or diminish emotional, physical, and spiritual suffering (Wright et al., 1996). To me, this talking about and listening to illness stories in purposeful therapeutic conversations become the context from which suffering can be alleviated and healing begins. I believe that cellular and "soulful" changes occur through these conversations. Our network of conversations and our relationships can contribute to the enhancement of diminishing pain experiences.

Suffering invites us into the spiritual domain. A shift to and emphasis on spirituality frequently represent the most profound response to suffering from chronic pain. If health professionals are to be helpful, we must acknowledge that suffer-

ing and, often, the senselessness of it are ultimately spiritual issues (Patterson, 1994).

The experience of suffering often becomes
transposed to one of spirituality when family
members try to make meaning out of their suffering and distress. Suffering leads one into the
spiritual domain as the big questions of life are
faced (Wright, 1999; Wright et al., 1996): questions such as, "Why has this illness happened to
me?" "Why do some people die before their
time?" or "What am I supposed to learn from
this suffering?" To understand how family members cope with suffering and what efforts can be
made to alleviate suffering, it is useful to explore
religious and spiritual beliefs in clinical work
with families.

Many beliefs and ideas exist about the purpose
of, lessons of, and reasons for suffering. The
medical perspective is that suffering occurs in response to pain and illness, as a response to the
meaning of symptoms, and when the impending
destruction of the person is perceived; and that
to remove the threat is to remove the suffering
(Morse, 2000).

Addressing the issue of what lessons can be
learned from suffering, Anne Morrow Lindbergh
writes:

 I do not believe that sheer suffering teaches. If
suffering alone taught, the entire world would be
wise since everyone suffers. To suffering must
be added mourning, understanding, patience,
love, openness and the willingness to remain
vulnerable.

Suffering and Theology

Theological perspectives suggest that suffering has redemptive and transformative qualities. For example, Whitney (1966) puts a more kindly face on suffering by suggesting certain benefits.

 No pain that we suffer, no trial that we experience is wasted. It ministers to our education, to the development of such qualities as patience, faith, fortitude and humility. All that we suffer and all that we endure, especially when we endure it patiently, builds up our characters, purifies our hearts, expands our souls, and makes us more tender and charitable. (p. 211)

Suffering does change us, and usually for the better. Frequently, we have a deepened compassion or a more tender heart or become less judgmental. But suffering can also invite bitterness over losses, confusion about life's abrupt changes, and anger over what might have been— even competitiveness over what type of suffering is the most severe.

Inattention to suffering may also be related to the perspective that many health professionals believe their purpose is to cure patients with the application of scientific knowledge, techniques, and skills. When a shift was made to thinking that disease had natural causes rather than supernatural sources, the spirit was separated from the body. In the traditional Christian outlook, both patients and their professional caregivers regarded suffering either as a consequence of one's own acts, and therefore to be endured; or as part of God's plan, to be accepted with the promise of a better existence in eternity. In this belief system, suffering had a religious and culturally defined interpretation (Reed, 2003).

The experience or depth of one person's suffering is never the same as someone else's. Suffering experiences cannot be compared, but unfortunately comparisons are made about which sufferings we believe are the most horrific. Is the breast cancer of a 33-year-old mother more devastating than the brain tumor of a 10-year-old boy? As Henri J.M. Nouwen (1996) so eloquently offers:

 I am deeply convinced that each human being suffers in a way no other human being suffers...in the final analysis, your pain and my pain are so deeply personal that comparing them can bring scarcely any consolation or comfort.

One philosophical belief frequently offered to those suffering with illness is that "life could be worse." This belief is offered to provide comfort and encouragement. One woman, suffering from endometriosis, did not find this belief useful, however. She responded, "I know life could be worse. I could have only one eye or leg, and I am very fortunate to have all I do have... But those philosophies do not solve the disease, do not get rid of the pain, the tears, the frustrations, or the heartaches that come with the problems" (Donoghue & Siegal, 1992, p. 55).

This particular suffering experience calls for nurses to recognize that each person's suffering is unique and that attempting to have persons

"count their blessings" can inadvertently trivialize suffering from illness.

Through highly privileged conversations between nurses and family members, it is readily
acknowledged that suffering, beliefs, and spirituality are close cousins (Wright, 1999). They are
so intertwined that it becomes difficult, or nearly
impossible, to discuss or attend to one without
attending to the others. (I have extended these
ideas even further and offered the theoretical
Trinity Model in Chapter 4.)

Suffering and Families

Suffering does not affect just the person experiencing an illness. Illness is a family affair, and all
family members suffer. If nurses would embrace
just this one belief—that illness is a family affair—it would change the face of nursing practice
(Wright & Leahey, 1999) and minimize suffering.
No one person in a family experiences cancer,
epilepsy, or heart disease. All family members
are influenced by the illness and, reciprocally, all
family members can contribute to the healing of
an illness.

On a personal note, if nurses had embraced
the belief that illness is a family affair and consequently that all family members suffer, it would
have provided much-needed healing for my family and me. During my mother's 5-year ordeal
with multiple sclerosis, she received competent
care from nurses, physicians, and other health
professionals for her physical suffering. But my
mother's emotional and spiritual suffering was

rarely addressed, and the suffering of my father, other family members, and myself was never addressed by nurses. During the last year of my mother's life, she had become a quadriplegic and experienced frequent severe pain in her hands. After one telephone call from my father, I was so struck by his words that I wrote them down. "We were having a great day until the pain returned—now nothing seems to be helping. I've given your mother all the pain medication, and more, that I can. I'm rubbing her hands with that new ointment. It's very tough to watch her suffer. I've lost my appetite and won't be having supper tonight; besides, I couldn't leave your mother alone in this pain." Is illness not a family affair? Who was suffering the most emotionally, my mother or my father? And who was suffering the most physically, or spiritually?

Morse and her colleagues in Canada have contributed much research effort to better understand the concept of suffering. One such study examined the concept of suffering and enduring and provided a framework that illustrated the interrelationships between these two distinct states (Morse & Carter, 1996). They identified a dynamic movement between enduring and suffering, dependent on the person's innate ability to handle the emotional work of suffering. Their study raised questions that could, from my perspective, be answered by examining actual clinical practice. For example, they raised the question, "What moves a person from enduring to suffering or from suffering back to enduring?" More recently, Morse and Penrod (1999) attempted to link the concepts of suffering, enduring, and uncertainty in the hope of constructing a comprehensive model for understanding and interpreting clinical situations.

Although all of these efforts can assist with our understanding of suffering, I believe that the best way to understand suffering is to examine conversations of ill sufferers and their nurses. Frank (2001) boldly suggests that:

 Too much research on illness rewrites their/our lives as behavior to be explained: coping, giving and receiving support, denial, adherence (the more politically correct name for the old compliance), even grieving all become behaviors to be explained as functional and adaptive with reference to clinically normative standards. (p. 16)

It might also be added that too much research on the behaviors of those who suffer may not alleviate but inadvertently contribute to suffering.

Therefore research needs to specify the beliefs and meanings of suffering so that these may be challenged to lessen suffering (Wright et al., 1996). Morse and Johnson (1991) also suggest that the primary goal should not only be to reduce the suffering of the ill person and/or the shared suffering but also to increase well-being!

Eifried (1998) conducted a hermeneutic-phenomenological study of nurses' lived experience of helping patients to find meaning during their experiences of suffering. Many of the themes reflected the same interventions designated as spiritual interventions in other studies—listening, being present, providing hope, calling forth voice, and being a guide. The author suggested that these "caring responses...are the foundation for spiritual nursing care" (p. 38), pointing to an understanding of care that embodies spirituality, rather than an understanding that nurses care for someone's spirit.

I believe that it is imperative that we connect the importance of intervention research with suffering. However, a nurse researcher immediately encounters significant challenges when embarking on research about suffering. How can the profound, human experience of suffering, particularly the suffering that accompanies serious illness, be fully appreciated and measured when examining interventions? What nursing behaviors can potentially enhance suffering? Perhaps the two most difficult questions for family nurse researchers are, "Can the profound experience of suffering be researched? (Frank, 2001) and, conversely, "Can research contribute to further suffering?"

Suffering and Family Nursing Interventions

If suffering is the center of nurses' clinical practice with families, what family nursing interventions are the most useful to assist families? What does current nursing research indicate about family nursing interventions that could contribute to the alleviation of suffering? What further research needs to be done? Family interventions in nursing are those healing practices that can diminish or alleviate suffering for individuals and families experiencing serious illness. Therefore intervention research should be the emphasis and focus of family nursing research (Wright & Bell, 1994).

To date, most research has revealed descriptions of the experience of suffering and what has NOT been done to alleviate suffering. In a study by Hinds (1992), the suffering of family caregivers of noninstitutionalized cancer patients revealed descriptions such as fear of loneliness, uncertainty about the future, communication breakdown, and lack of support.

Spouses of women receiving chemotherapy reported suffering themselves during their partners' illness (Wilson, 1991). As these husbands struggled to buffer their wives from the effects of chemotherapy, they also struggled to maintain control of their own feelings of helplessness. They perceived that they were "kept in the dark" and had the perception that the lack of communication with their wives and with health-care providers increased their feelings of helplessness and powerlessness; ultimately, the suffering of these husbands increased. Some of the husbands wished they had been able to talk to someone else, particularly an outsider, and they recognized that remaining silent had impeded their ability to cope with the cancer experience.

What are possible answers to the most difficult questions for nurse researchers and clinicians mentioned previously: can the profound experience of suffering be researched? (Frank, 2001). Can research contribute to further suffering?

Frank (2001) argues that some aspects of suffering remain unspeakable. However, I believe the aspects of suffering that can be spoken of may be lessened when there is acknowledgment of, witnessing, or "just listening" (Frank, 1998) to the ill person. For suffering to be lessened, nurses must be willing to encounter suffering with ill persons and their family members. Engagement and suffering are essential aspects of responsible caregiving (Schultz & Carnevale, 1996).

Suffering can be researched without contributing further to an individual's suffering if we fully engage with our clients and family members who are living with suffering. Wilson (1991) asks this poignant question in reporting her research, "How does the researcher listen to such suffering and remain detached?" I submit that remaining detached does not allow one to know, understand, or research another's suffering.

Why would we, as nurse researchers, clinicians, or educators, want to remain detached from another's suffering? I am familiar with the arguments that researchers offer about the need to remain detached and distant from the topic and subjects being researched. Could our research not take on a more human and humane dimension if we allowed ourselves to be touched and moved by suffering?

My colleagues, Drs. Wendy L. Watson and Janice M. Bell, and I evolved a clinical approach, namely the Illness Beliefs Model, to working with families in which a member is seriously ill (Wright et al., 1996). We emphasize altering, challenging, or modifying constraining beliefs as one way to assist with alleviating or diminishing suffering in families. Some of the ways we have found useful in alleviating suffering are acknowledging suffering; inviting stories of, listening to, and witnessing suffering; connecting suffering and spirituality; recognizing and challenging our own constraining beliefs; creating a healing environment; and inviting reflections about suffering (Wright, 1999; Wright et al., 1996). (See Chapter 5 for an in-depth discussion for creating a context for conversations of suffering and spirituality.)

For example, what influence or connection do illness beliefs have in relation to suffering, and vice versa? What influence or connection do family members' and nurses' notions of spirituality have on their suffering? The potential contribution of this type of research is to continue advancing our knowledge about living with and suffering from serious illness. If we have a better understanding of what aspects of these conversations can potentially heal suffering, the importance of routinely inviting these conversations of suffering and involving family members in health care can be further advocated and admonished.

This type of research will also point the direction for the necessary knowledge and skills required by nurses to assist in the very ethical and obligatory endeavor of assisting individuals and family members who suffer with serious illness. This is one example of the kind of research that moves beyond defining and describing *suffering.* It is time to research what specific nursing interventions in our conversations of suffering create the conditions for healing to occur.

In our clinical work in the Family Nursing Unit (FNU) at the University of Calgary, we believe that creating a trusting environment for therapeutic conversations invites open expression of family members' fears, anger, and sadness about their illness experiences (Wright et al., 1996). By creating a trusting environment for the expression of strong affect, we can contribute to the reduction of suffering. (See Chapter 5 for an embellished discussion of clinical ideas that assist in reducing or eliminating suffering.)

Previous family nursing research studies conducted within the FNU are beginning to illuminate what particular family nursing interventions are healing and therefore reduce suffering. Robinson's (1994) study examined the process and outcomes of interventions with families experiencing chronic illness. Her study revealed: "... two major components of therapeutic change from the families' perspective are: creating the circumstances for change and moving beyond/ overcoming problems" (p. 99). Specifically, the nurses' acts of bringing the family together and creating a sense of comfort and trust were the fundamental behaviors that enabled family members to convey their illness experiences. Providing a context for sharing illness experiences with family members legitimizes the intense emotions generated by these experiences. Expressing the impact of the illness on the family and, reciprocally, the influence of the family on the illness gives validation and voice to the experiences and thereby are healing practices that reduce suffering.

Tapp (1997; 2001) explored the therapeutic conversations between nurses and families experiencing ischemic heart disease within the FNU. These therapeutic conversations moved beyond social conversations and were purposeful, deliberate, and healing. She discovered that the conversations between nurses and families were about healthy lifestyles, family support, uncertainty, and death. When spaces were created for these therapeutic conversations, conditions emerged for healing to occur. When nurses engaged in these particular types of conversations with families experiencing heart disease, suffering was diminished as possibilities for making sense of the illness and suffering were revealed.

A qualitative study by Moules (2000; 2002) explored the use of therapeutic letters within the clinical practice at the FNU. Her thoughtful and illuminating findings suggest that therapeutic letters written by nurses and mailed to families after family meetings have the potential for further healing and minimizing of suffering. Houger Limacher (2003) contributed to our knowledge by conducting research to further understand the family systems nursing intervention of "commendations" (Wright et al., 1996). Commending patients and family members on their strengths, resources, and competencies in the midst of illness, asking reflective questions, and expanding the therapeutic relationship all serve to create a context for healing. But Houger Limacher suggests, and I believe, that it is the "goodness" embedded in commendations that invites healing.

McLeod's (2003) hermeneutic inquiry undertaken to explore the meaning of spirituality and spiritual care practices in family systems nursing, also a first of its kind, suggests that suffering embodies an obligation to respond to the spiritual.

All of the aforementioned studies of particular nursing practices and interventions are revealing and bring forth conversations of suffering, thereby acknowledging that suffering exists. These research studies conducted within the FNU strongly suggest that it is not just a good thing or a nice thing to provide opportunities for families to have conversations about their suffering, but that it is necessary and imperative if healing is to occur!

Nurses must have as their primary goal the creation of an environment for alleviating and/or healing emotional, physical, and spiritual suffering (Wright, 1997, 1999; Wright et al., 1996).

Presentations and Publications about Suffering

In our presentations and publications, we must truly honor those who suffer with illness and who graciously participate in our research studies. We can do this through our tone, affect, and manner in our presentations and publications and by demonstrating the congruence between the research findings and our response to them.

We must ensure that those who suffer from illness and their family members have not gone unheard. We can do this by acknowledging and affirming that we have been touched and softened by those who suffer. Research about how to comfort and heal those who are suffering must not matter just in the moment of a conference presentation or a professional publication; it must also matter in our nursing practice.

Research that addresses illness addresses suffering. Therefore our research findings, conclusions, reflections, and discoveries must illuminate suffering and how to heal, diminish, or alleviate it. Most important, our research findings must be offered in a manner that will be taken up in nursing practice. We hope that nurse researchers who examine interventions used with individuals and families will become more committed and attuned to the marvelous potential their research studies possess for healing. And from the research process and findings, nurses in practice can use the ideas from the findings and add new ideas that we can reaffirm to reclaim our desire and motivation to be healers to those who suffer.

The dearth of scholarship about suffering in patient care is evidenced in the fact that major health-care texts and bibliographical databases, such as MEDLINE, contain few citations about suffering (Reed, 2003). Reed (2003) further suggests that those that do exist tend to equate suffering with physiological pain or to treat it as an indicator of disease or a secondary focus or illness. I concur with Reed (2003) that there is no agreed-on theory of suffering in the literature, or any premises that lead to a consistent or common definition of suffering. However, it is my hope that this text will add one more voice to the efforts of professionals, particularly nurses, who attempt to study, understand, and alleviate suffering! I trust that the most useful contributions of this book are the actual clinical examples with individuals and families whereby my clinical team and I attempt to alleviate or diminish their suffering.

References

Donoghue, P.J., & Siegel, M.E. (1992). *Sick and tired of feeling sick and tired: Living with invisible chronic illness*. New York: Norton.

Eifried, S. (1998). Helping patients find meaning: A caring response to suffering. *International Journal of Caring, 2*(1), 33–39.

Frank, A. (1998). Just listening: Narrative and deep illness. *Families, Systems, and Health, 16*(3), 197–212.

Frank, A. (2001). Can we research suffering? *Qualitative Health Research, 11*(3), 353–362.

Frank, A.W. (1994). Interrupted stories, interrupted lives. *Second Opinion, 20*(1), 11–18.

Frank, A.W. (1995). *The Wounded Storyteller: Body, Illness, and Ethics*. Chicago: University of Chicago Press.

Hinds, C. (1992). Suffering: A relatively unexplored phenomena among family caregivers of non-institutionalized patients with cancer. *Journal of Advanced Nursing, 17*, 918–925.

Houger Limacher, L. (2003). Commendations: The healing potential of one family systems nursing intervention. Unpublished doctoral thesis: University of Calgary, Calgary, Alberta, Canada.

Kleinman, D. (1988). *The illness narrative.* New York: Basic Books.

Lindholm, L., & Eriksson, K. (1993). To understand and alleviate suffering in a caring culture. *Journal of Advanced Nursing, 18,* 1354–1361.

McLeod, D.L. (2003). Opening space for the spiritual: Therapeutic conversations with families living with serious illness. Unpublished doctoral thesis, University of Calgary, Alberta, Canada.

Morse, J. (2000). The idiosyncrasies of self-being. Presented at the International Qualitative Heath Research Conference, April, Banff, Canada.

Morse, J.M., & Carter, B.J. (1996). The essence of enduring and the expression of suffering: The re-formulation of self. *Scholarly Inquiry for Nursing Practice, 10*(1), 43–60.

Morse, J.M., & Johnson, J.L. (1991). Toward a theory of illness: The Illness-Constellation Model. In J.M. Morse & J.L. Johnson (Eds.), *The illness experience: Dimensions of suffering* (pp. 315–342). Newbury Park, CA: Sage.

Morse, J.M., & Penrod, J. (1999). Linking concepts of enduring, uncertainty, suffering, and hope. *Image: Journal of Nursing Scholarship, 31*(2), 145–150.

Moules, N.J. (2000). Nursing on paper: The art and mystery of therapeutic letters in clinical work with families experiencing illness. Unpublished doctoral dissertation, University of Calgary, Alberta, Canada.

Moules, N.J. (2002). Nursing on paper: Therapeutic letters in nursing practice. *Nursing Inquiry, 9*(2), 104–113.

Nouwen, H.J.M. (1996). *Can you drink this cup?* (p. 35) Notre Dame, Illinois: Ava Maria Press.

Patterson, R.B. (1994, June). Learning from suffering. *Family Therapy News*, pp. 11–12.

Reed, F.C. (2003). *Suffering and illness: Insights for caregivers*. Philadelphia: F.A. Davis Co.

Robinson, C.A. (1994). *Women, families, chronic illness and nursing interventions: From burden to balance*. Unpublished doctoral dissertation, University of Calgary, Alberta, Canada.

Robinson, C.A., & Wright, L.M. (1995). Family nursing interventions: What families say makes a difference. *Journal of Family Nursing, 1*(3), 327–345.

Schultz, D.S., & Carnevale, F. (1996). Engagement and suffering in responsible caregiving: On overcoming maleficence in health care. *Theoretical Medicine, 17*, 189–207.

Tapp, D.M. (2001). Conserving the vitality of suffering: Addressing family constraints to illness conversations. *Nursing Inquiry, 8*(4), 254–263.

Tapp, D.M. (1997). Exploring therapeutic conversations between nurses and families experiencing ischemic heart disease. Unpublished doctoral dissertation, University of Calgary, Alberta, Canada.

Whitney, O.F. (1966). Suffering. *Improvement Era*, March, 210–212.

Wilson, S. (1991). The unrelenting nightmare: Husbands' experiences during their wives' chemotherapy. In J.M. Morse & J.L. Johnson (Eds.), *The illness experience: Dimensions of suffering* (pp. 237–314). Newbury Park, CA: Sage.

Wright, L.M. (1999). Spirituality, suffering and beliefs: The soul of healing with families. In F. Walsh

(Ed.). *Spiritual resources in family therapy* (pp. 61–75). New York: Guilford Press.

Wright, L.M. (1997). Multiple sclerosis, beliefs, and families: Professional and personal stories of suffering and strength. In S. McDaniel, J. Hepworth, & W.J. Doherty (Eds.), *The shared experience of illness: Stories of patients, families, and their therapists* (pp. 263–273). New York: Basic Books.

Wright, L.M., & Bell, J.M. (1994). The future of family nursing research: Interventions, interventions, interventions. *The Japanese Journal of Nursing Research, 27*(2–3), 4–15.

Wright, L.M., & Leahey, M. (1999). Maximizing time, minimizing suffering: The 15 minute (or less) family interview. *Journal of Family Nursing, 5*(3), 259–273.

Wright, L.M., Watson, W.L., & Bell, J.M. (1996). *Beliefs: The heart of healing in families and illness*. New York: Basic Books.

3

Spirituality and Illness in Professional Literature

Deborah L. McLeod

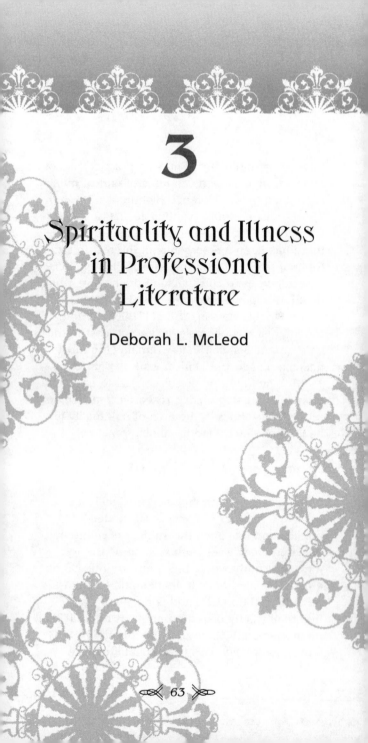

Interest in spirituality in nursing practices is not new, having existed as an integral part of nursing since long before Florence Nightingale (Barnum, 1996; Nelson, 2000; Nightingale, 1859/1969; O'Brien, 1999). However, over recent decades, there has been a resurgence of interest in the topic of spirituality on the part of theoreticians, researchers, and clinicians in nursing and other health disciplines (Barnum, 1996; O'Brien, 1999; Wright, Watson, & Bell, 1996). Although the interest has been significant, at least in the care of families, spirituality remains the most neglected aspect of clinical work (Wright et al., 1996). The following discussion explores the literature of nursing theory, research, practice, and related disciplines in the area of spirituality in health and illness and in nursing practice.

Theorizing Spirituality

Spirituality has been included in significant ways in a number of conceptual models of nursing and has been the subject of numerous conceptual analyses. Although some theory may be useful, overall this literature reflects our empirical inheritance in its demand for, and pursuit of, theoretical and conceptual clarity. Spirituality is theorized primarily as an individual phenomenon, with virtually no attention to family spirituality. This theoretical literature is reviewed, critiqued, and extended in the following sections.

Remembering Spirituality

Until the mid-20th century, nursing had been associated with, or actually existed under the auspices of, religious institutions. Nursing practice has therefore been strongly influenced by religious ideals, particularly an ethic of "doing good" and taking care of those who are suffering (O'Brien, 1999). Florence Nightingale, the mother of modern nursing, theorized about the spiritual focus of nursing practice. Nightingale believed that she was "called" by God to serve humanity. To contribute to the development of a sense of spiritual well-being in her patients, Nightingale focused on developing "sympathy," a concept similar to the idea of empathy. Sympathy was understood as a mode for shared experience with others that included the idea of tolerance for others' beliefs and religious practices (Widerquist, 1992).

Gradually, however, as the natural sciences became the preferred way of understanding everything related to the body, nursing's spiritual and religious sensibilities became submerged in the Cartesian discourse that dominated the scientific curricula of nursing schools throughout the first half of the 20th century. Secular views were separated from sacred morals and physical reality from spiritual being (Brittain, 1986). By the 1960s, illness was considered strictly a pathophysiological event (Keegan, 1994), and the majority of nursing schools were no longer associated with religious institutions.

The overt religious commitments of nursing have been left behind, at least as far as the academic nursing discourse is concerned. The residues of nursing's religious sensibilities have been subsumed in the current topic of interest, spirituality. The nursing literature of the past few decades suggests that spiritual issues have been neglected in actual nursing practice, as well as in nursing theory and research. This acknowledgment seems to have sparked renewed interest in the research and theory of spirituality and spiritual care, particularly in regard to individuals (Barnum, 1996; Dyson, Cobb, & Forman, 1997; Laukhuf & Werner, 1998; Tuck, Pullen, & Wallace, 2001), but also, to a lesser extent, with families (Marshall et al., 2003; Wright et al., 1996). Far more of this literature has been centered in academic thought, whereas far less has been grounded in the actual practices of nurses, contributing to a proliferation of literature that has little meaning to clinicians and that provides little grounding for care. The meaning of spirituality in nursing practice continues to be poorly articulated (Cusveller, 1998; Martsolf & Mickley, 1998). Similar acknowledgment and interest have been seen in medicine (Benson, 1996; Dossey, 1993; Koenig, McCullough, & Larson, 2001; Kristeller, Zumbrun, & Schilling, 1999; Larson, 1993; Mathews, Larson, & Barry, 1993), psychology (Bergin, 1991; Richards & Bergin, 1997), sociology (Ellison & Levin, 1998), and family therapy (Anderson & Worthen, 1997;

Becvar, 1996; Carlson & Erickson, 2002; Carlson, Kirkpatrick, Hecker, & Killmer, 2002; Chubb, Gutsche, & Efron, 1994; Griffith & Griffith, 2002; Prest & Keller, 1993; Stewart & Gale, 1994; Walsh, 1999).

The inclusion of nursing responsibility for spiritual care cited by the International Council of Nurses in their Code of Ethics by the American Holistic Nurses Association in their Standards for Holistic Nursing Practice, and through the development of a nursing diagnostic category, Spiritual Distress, by the North American Nursing Diagnosis Association (NANDA) (Hall & Lanig, 1993) speaks to the increased interest in spirituality in nursing. Barnum (1996) has attributed this increased attention, in part, to the growth of the discourse of "holistic" nursing practice. In addition, however, research on religious and spiritual topics has become more "respectable" in recent years, with the burgeoning research evidence that spirituality and religion do make a positive difference in health and illness (Ellison & Levin, 1998; Larson, 2001; Richards & Bergin, 1997). The general public in North America has also demonstrated increasing interest in spirituality, although not particularly in traditional religious institutions (Bibby, 1987, 1993, 2002; Elkins, 1999; Swenson, 1999), possibly adding further impetus to health-care practitioners to consider the relevance of spirituality in health care.

Within the area of marriage and family therapy, there is perhaps one additional contribution to the increased interest in spirituality. During the past decade, marriage and family therapists have become much more attuned to issues of diversity such as gender and cultural diversity (Bird, 2000; White & Tapping, 1990). Religion and spirituality represent one more aspect of diversity in psychotherapy that is beginning to garner attention (Adams, 1995; Bergin, 1991; Boyd-Franklin & Lockwood, 1999; Lukoff, Lu, & Turner, 1992; Stewart & Gale, 1994).

The Spiritual Dimensions of Persons

The view of the person that includes a spiritual dimension has emerged in contemporary conceptual models of nursing, particularly in the work of Jean Watson (1988), Margaret Newman (1994), Betty Neuman (1995), and Barbara Dossey (Dossey, Keegan, Guzzetta, Kolkmeirer, 1995). Although each of these models is very different in focus, all four models strongly support the notion that spirituality is an integral part of understanding human beings, health, and nursing practice.

The idea of a person as continuously growing and developing often connects to the idea of growing toward a higher good (such as God). In Watson's (1988) conception of *person*, the notion of *spirit* reflects this goal orientation, as does Newman's (1994), albeit in different language. Neuman (1995) understood a person as being animated through his or her spirit and that spirituality permeates all aspects of a person, regardless of whether it is acknowledged or developed. For Dossey and her colleagues (1995), spirituality was understood as having three defining characteristics. The first characteristic, *unfolding mystery*, refers to one's experiences of life's meaning and purpose. The second, *inner strengths*, refers to self, consciousness, transcendence, and both inner and sacred resources. The third characteristic, *harmonious interconnectedness*, refers to interconnections with self, others, a higher power or God, and the environment (Dossey et al., 1995, p. 22). These authors differentiated nursing care as either *doing*, such as medications and procedures, or *being*, which includes such as things as imagery, prayer, meditation, and quiet contemplation, as well as the presence and intention of the nurse.

In addition to the formal conceptual models of nursing, much effort has gone into defining and conceptualizing *spirituality* as a phenomenon of interest. A number of authors (Burkhardt, 1989, 1994; Cusveller, 1998; Emblen, 1992; Martsolf & Mickley, 1998; McSherry & Draper, 1998; Oldnall, 1995; Reed, 1992) suggested that it is important to differentiate between religion and spirituality. They make the assumption that distinction, definition, and clarity will contribute to the integration of spiritual care in nursing practices. Spirituality is generally portrayed in the literature as a broader, more inclusive concept than religion (Dyson et al., 1997; Nagai-Jacobson

& Burkhardt, 1989; Wright et al., 1996).
Burkhardt (1989) viewed spirituality as a unifying force or vital principle of a person that integrates all other aspects of human beings. One understanding of spirituality is that it is:

 ... a belief in and experience of a supreme being or an ultimate human condition, along with an internal set of values and active investment in those values, a sense of connection, a sense of meaning, and a sense of inner wholeness. (MacKinnon et al., 1994, as cited in Wright et al., 1996, p. 30)

In her literature review of the concept, Fry (1998) suggests that the range of definitions of spirituality includes those related to personal transcendence, interpersonal relationships, the transpersonal realm, and all three. Barnum (1996) found that, in some nursing literature, spirituality has been associated with a traditional religious context; in others, with an advanced level of human development; and in still others, with growth beyond insular human existence. Because most of the theories that consider spirituality are holistic in nature, spirituality has become associated with *holism,* the etymological roots of which mean "holy" (Newman, 1994).

Emblen (1992) surveyed more than 30 years of the nursing literature to distinguish the concept of religion from that of spirituality through the use of concept analysis procedures. The following nine words appeared in defining spirituality: *personal, life, principle, animator, being, God, quality, relationship,* and *transcendent.*

Six words were associated with religion: *systems, beliefs, organized, person, worship,* and *practices.* Emblen concluded that the terms reflect distinct concepts that exist in relationship to each other. In analyzing the concept of spirituality emerging in nursing literature, Martsolf and Mickley (1998) identified the following attributes of spirituality: *meaning, value, transcendence, connecting,* and *becoming.* Religion, however, has been understood as referring to a system of institutionalized beliefs that involve shared values and beliefs about God, the Divine, or some other higher principle. More recent analyses have reported similar findings (Tanyi, 2002). Religion also implies involvement with a community that shares those beliefs and values (Wright et al., 1996).

The etymological roots of *spirit* include the Latin *pneuma,* meaning "soul," "courage," "vigor," and "breath." *Spirit* is also derived from the Hebrew *ruach* and the Greek *pneuma,* both of which also point to "breath" or "breath of life" (Barnhart, 1988).

A related term, "soul," is explored in a helpful piece entitled, "The salvation of your souls: But what is a soul?" (Carter, 2000), which traced the etymological roots, in part, to the Old English *sawl. Sawl* is also the root for the word "sea," which was believed to be the place of habitation of souls in Celtic mythology. Symbols of the soul have always been related to nature and include such images as the wind, the sea, and water. Although language varies, all cultures seem to have some conception of the soul as a center of being. In the Dani culture of New Guinea, for example, all creatures except reptiles and insects are believed to possess a soul called *etai-eken,* or "seeds of singing" (Carter, 2000). Augustine identified three aspects of soul, one of which was *pneuma* ("spirit"). The terms "spirit" and "soul," for some, have come to be used interchangeably, although within the health-care literature, the term "spirit" is used much more commonly. In other cases (Anderson, 1999; Moore, 1992/1994, 1994; Smucker, 1996), however, *soul* continues to be interpreted as one aspect of spirit. In this understanding, soul is tied to the body and mind, including thought, action, and emotion. Soul relates to the immanence, rather than the transcendence, of spirit, to "genuine community, and attachment to the world" (Moore, 1992/1994, p. 229).

Although many nurses have placed emphasis on differentiating spirituality from religion, it may be important to keep in mind the findings of one study (Joanides, 1997) that explored the meaning of spirituality and religion with a group of Orthodox Christians. For this population, drawing distinctions between the terms was not useful or congruent with their understandings of spirituality/religion. The participants in this study considered the terms to be inseparable and could not relate to requests to differentiate these. Joanides (1997) concluded that insisting on separation might contribute to clinicians inadvertently limiting conversations with families because of different understandings and biases about terminology. Similarly, in her analysis of a number of case studies, Mayer (1992) found that in the practice of spiritual care, neither nurses nor patients struggled with ambiguity about the terms "spirituality" and "religion." Perhaps the struggle with clarity and definition reflects the effort to study spirituality using the methods of the natural sciences, a predominant approach in the health-care literature.

Thomas Matus, a Benedictine monk, in conversation with Fritjof Capra and David Steindl-Rast (1991), offered some thoughts about the relationship between religion and spirituality:

 You can have spirituality without religion, but you cannot have religion, authentic religion, without spirituality... . So the priority belongs...to spirituality as experience, a direct knowledge of absolute Spirit in the here and now, and as praxis, a knowledge that transforms the way I live out my life in this world... . Institutionalization is one of the consequences when an original spiritual experience is transformed into a religion...religion brings out the intellectual dimension of spirituality, when it seeks to understand and express the original experience in words and concepts; and then it brings out the social dimension, when it makes the experience a principle of life and action for a community. (pp. 12–13)

To consider religion and spirituality as *praxis*, transforming the living of life, highlights the relationship between them and may add a useful dimension to our understanding. In general, religion can be understood to be the language of the spiritual, which attempts to explain or describe the spiritual; spirituality itself is, according to Steindl-Rast, experience. It has a language of its own that does not readily translate and is different from human language.

Moore (1992/1994) suggested that there were two ways of thinking about religion. He suggested that the church allows us to be in the presence of the holy, to contemplate, and to be influenced by that presence. Religion also teaches us to see the sacred dimension of everyday life, both directly and symbolically. Religion is, in Moore's reading of it, an "art of memory" and a way of being mindful of the sacred.

The foregoing discussion perhaps highlights the difficulties in resolving the ambiguity of both the terminology of, and the relationship between, spirituality and religion. Clearly, there is a tension between the two that may be more important to attend to than to resolve through definition. The effort to differentiate terms seems motivated by both the requirements of natural science methodologies and the assumption that clarity will increase nurses' ability to integrate spirituality in their practices. This also reflects an interpretation of *nursing* as an applied science, in which *theory* is understood to direct practice (Bishop & Scudder, 1995). Although some clarity is needed, too much may contribute to *rigidity*, a closing down rather than an opening up of spirituality to understanding.

Toward an Understanding of a Family Spirituality

Conceptual models of nursing rarely address the family as client, implying the inclusion of family in the general concept of client. In many respects this is unsatisfactory because a family is very different than an individual client, for whom these models seem to be written.

One theme reflected in the theoretical literature is that relationships are an integral part of one's experience of spirituality. In some ways, then, it is strange that spirituality is taken up almost without exception in the nursing literature as an individual phenomenon, with such limited acknowledgment of the social and environmental aspects. Perhaps this reflects the neglect of families, communities, and the environment more generally in nursing and health care, which tends to be strongly individualistic. However, if spirituality is understood to be about meaning that occurs in relationship with others, the family becomes key to both the experience and practice of spirituality. This is particularly so when one understands *family* as "a group of individuals who are bound by strong emotional ties, a sense of belonging, and a passion for being involved in one another's lives" (Wright et al., 1996, p. 45). As others have suggested, "faith is inherently relational, from our earliest years, when the most fundamental convictions about life are shaped within caregiving relationships" (Walsh, 1999, p. 22).

Religious and spiritual beliefs are among the most powerful beliefs we hold and contribute significantly to ways of making sense of the world (Wright et al., 1996). A *belief* is understood to be a persisting set of premises about what is taken to be true (Wright et al., 1996) and is forged in community, socially constructed in language within our families and the larger community (Anderson & Goolishian, 1988; Hoffman, 1990, Wright et al., 1996). Our beliefs are an ingredient in the glue of family and larger community:

 Beliefs distinguish one person from another, yet also join people together. Through our living and being together, we influence each other's beliefs. We develop our identities within our families, professions, and communities through the belief systems that we share and do not share with others. We live our lives only slightly aware, and sometimes not at all aware, of our beliefs and the effect they have on our own lives and the lives of others. (Wright et al., 1996, pp. 19–20)

Family rituals are important avenues for the development, sharing, evolving, and passing on to future generations the belief systems that are of most importance to a family. Rituals are often religious in nature, including such things as weddings, funerals, and family prayer times. Family belief systems and their expression in ritual (formal and elaborate; informal and simple) provide a way of making sense out of life events (Imber-Black, Roberts, & Whiting, 1993; Walsh, 1999), allowing us to preserve and enrich the spirituality embodied in relationships.

Anderson (1999) suggests that the renewal of an embodied family spirituality demands that we examine the metaphors that we use to think about the human person. The label of the *self* suggests a social construction, whereas the idea of person as a biopsychosocial spiritual being is more captured in the label *soul*. Soul thrives on a spirituality that is not only transcendent but also grounded in the spirit of the family, linked to generations of traditions, values, and stories. *Stories* are the memories of a family and a people; "it is memory that makes our lives personally meaningful by linking the past and the present...when we have lost our memory, we have also lost our soul" (Anderson, 1999, p. 159). Offering a place for families to tell stories provides opportunities to claim memory and soul. Within the practice of family nursing, "the inviting, listening to, and witnessing of illness stories provide a powerful validation of a profound human experience" (Wright, 1999, p. 67). Such validation might be understood as soul care.

The Research Literature: Spirituality and Illness

Substantial bodies of literature are accumulating that attest to the importance of spiritual and religious variables in health and illness (Benson, 1996; Dossey, 1993; Ellison & Levin, 1998; Gartner, 1996; Koenig, 1995; Koenig et al., 2001; Mathews et al., 1993; Mickley, Carson, & Soeken, 1995; Weaver, Flannelly, Flannelly,

Koenig, & Larson, 1998). In addition to the literature examining these relationships, there has been considerable interest in nursing in the study of spiritual needs and spiritual care (Barnum, 1996; Carson, 1989; Hermann, 2001; O'Brien, 1999). However, with few exceptions (Stiles, 1990), there has been very little research about spirituality in family nursing, family systems nursing, or family therapy (Wright, 1999).

In the medical literature, which is largely American in origin, the preferred terminology and focus of study is "religion." This terminology is more reflective of the beliefs of American researchers, most of whom are religious and identify more with the idea of "religion" than "spirituality." However, much of the literature *has* only looked at "religion," not spirituality, by measuring such variables as church affiliation and attendance (Ellison & Levin, 1998; Koenig et al., 2001; Larson, 2001). Even in recent literature (Ellison & Levin, 1998), the call for future research is to focus on differentiating the "behavioral" (e.g., church attendance, prayer) from the "functional" (health behaviors, social ties, coping strategies) aspects of religious involvement, not on spirituality.

In sharp contrast, the favored term in nursing is almost exclusively spirituality. This perhaps reflects the efforts in nursing to theorize about the nature of human beings, and nursing understands persons as biopsychosocial-spiritual beings to a much greater degree than do some other disciplines.

Relationships between Religion and Health

A large body of research, largely associated with disciplines other than nursing such as medicine and psychology, has focused on the relationship between religion and some health-related outcome. Although the language of "health outcomes" is used, many of the studies really examined "disease outcomes." Positive relationships between religion, often defined as church attendance and affiliation (although sometimes defined as spiritual well-being), and a wide variety of disease and health outcomes have been identified. Although small to modest, this relationship seems relatively consistent across studies, despite limitations in measurement (Ellison & Levin, 1998; Koenig et al., 2001). Epidemiological studies of mortality and overall health, including some longitudinal studies, have documented these effects, and both physical and mental diseases have been examined. Examples of physical disease conditions that have been studied include cardiovascular disorders such as hypertension, coronary artery disease, and strokes, as well as cancer, immune system disorders, and a variety of symptoms such as disability and pain. In addition, relationships have been studied with mental health disorders such as depression, anxiety, suicidality, substance abuse, and schizophrenia. The consensus is that, although many of the studies in the past were limited by homogeneous samples,

cross-sectional designs, and inadequate measures of religious variables, more recent studies
that overcome these limitations continue to
show a positive relationship (Ellison & Levin,
1998; Koenig et al., 2001).

Koenig and colleagues (2001) suggest the
need to examine possible negative effects of religion and call for more longitudinal and intervention studies in a number of areas. The most
pressing need, they suggest, however, is related
to the integration of knowledge into clinical practice. The proposed research trajectories imply
that knowledge will be integrated into practice
through the eventual testing (using randomized
controlled trials) of interventions that manipulate
religious practices and experiences for the benefit of one's health. It is difficult to imagine, however, that the instrumental use of sacred
practices and experiences would be acceptable
for many religious persons, or even possible.
Nonetheless, this body of research has clearly
demonstrated the health benefits of religious
practices, confirming the importance of health
professionals incorporating at least a respect for
this aspect of life into their practices.

Nursing Research and Spirituality

Within nursing, research has focused on health-
related outcomes, identification of spiritual
needs and spiritual care, and interpretations of
the lived experience of spirituality for persons

and nurses. Although the language is more consistently about spirituality than about religion, many of the studies do use measures of religiosity. As might be expected in nursing, the health outcomes examined tend to emphasize issues related to illness, rather than disease, including such outcomes as coping and quality of life.

HEALTH OUTCOMES AND SPIRITUALITY

There is a substantial body of empirical nursing research in the context of chronic and life-threatening illness that reveals a positive relationship between spiritual and religious variables and a wide variety of health-related outcomes. Some recent examples of studies examining the relationship between religious/spiritual variables and outcomes include the following: feelings of health and well-being (Fehring, Miller, & Shaw, 1997; Fryback & Reinert, 1999; Kurtz, Wyatt, & Kurtz, 1995), coping (Feher & Maly, 1999; Fredette, 1995), quality of life (Ferrell et al., 1996; Wyatt & Friedman, 1996), meaning and hope (Ballard, Green, McCaa, & Logsdon, 1997; Feher & Maly, 1999; Fryback & Reinert, 1999), social support (Feher & Maly, 1999), and demands of illness (Fernsler, Klemm, & Miller, 1999).

This body of literature is not without difficulties. As in other disciplines, most of the above studies are correlational in design, limiting the conclusions you might draw. Spiritual and religious variables for the most part are operationally defined and measured using existing instruments that are valid and reliable. However, many of the instruments have been criticized for not being culturally relevant for some (Mytko & Knight, 1999) and for reflecting a strong Judeo-Christian bias. Although there are limitations, the findings across studies demonstrate the positive influence of spiritual and religious dimensions of life for health and well-being in the context of serious illness.

In addition to the empirical studies, there are accumulating numbers of studies guided by qualitative and interpretive approaches that also support the importance of spirituality in health and as a resource in illness and healing (Burkhardt, 1994; Chiu, 2000; Smucker, 1996; Stiles, 1990; Walton, 1999).

SPIRITUAL NEEDS

There is an emphasis on the identification, or "assessment," of spiritual needs in both the theoretical and research literature (Barnum, 1996; Carson, 1989; Hermann, 2001; O'Brien, 1999; Stoll, 1979). Spiritual needs are conceived as the need to find meaning in the midst of illness and suffering; the need to affirm relationships to self, others, God, and nature; and the need for the realization of transcendent values such as hope and creativity, compassion, faith, peace, trust, courage, and love (Emblen & Halstead, 1993; Highfield and Cason, 1983; O'Brien, 1999).

In response to the question, "What needs can you identify related to your spirituality as you describe it?" older hospice patients identified 29 different spiritual needs (Hermann, 2001). These needs were clustered under six themes: religious practices, companionship, involvement and control, finishing business, experiencing nature, and having a positive outlook. According to Hermann (2001), "Nurses must be able to identify patients' specific spiritual needs to intervene" (p. 68).

Related to spiritual needs is the nursing diagnosis of Spiritual Distress, identified by NANDA. *Spiritual distress* is defined by NANDA as a "disruption in the life principle which pervades a person's entire being and which integrates and transcends one's biological and psychological nature" (Kim, McFarland, & McLane, 1987, p. 55). This diagnostic category has influenced nurses to attend more to assessment and the development of interventions in the area of spirituality (Burnard, 1987; Emblen & Halstead, 1993), resulting in assessment frameworks (Dossey et al., 1995) and models (Emblen & Pesut, 2001).

Research on spiritual needs clearly reflects a desire for theory that will allow control and prediction and a belief that once needs are clearly identified, nurses will be able to intervene. This approach can invite rigid thinking or only the understanding of nursing as an applied science or a technology. Mayer (1992) suggested that conceiving of persons as a collection of needs is simply a popular way of parceling out aspects of a life to the appropriate "experts" who are in the business of meeting them. Defining spirituality in terms of spiritual needs also invites a view of spirituality as a cluster of problems that by definition require a solution.

SPIRITUAL CARE PRACTICES

The literature reflects a relative consistency across studies about the nature of nursing interventions for spiritual needs. Interventions include those that involve "doing" (such as prayer, referral, physical care, alleviation of pain, creation of an environment that provides for spiritual or religious practices) as well as "being" (listening, being with, sharing, supporting, respecting, compassion), to borrow Dossey et al.'s (1995) terminology.

One study (Clarke, Cross, Deane, & Lowry, 1991) explored the perceptions of spiritual care of 15 previously hospitalized adult patients. In a structured interview, participants were asked about which hospital experiences contributed to hope and well-being and which negatively affected recovery, as well as what might have been done to further enhance their sense of well-being during the hospitalization. The authors conclude with a recommendation for five spiritual interventions: (1) establishing a trusting relationship, (2) providing and facilitating a supportive environment, (3) responding sensitively to patients' beliefs, (4) integrating spirituality into the quality assurance plan, and (5) taking ownership of the nurse's key role in the health-care system. Barnum (1996) suggests that perhaps these interventions could simply be related to good psychological care (or just good care) without necessarily being about spirituality. However, the list reflects that "spiritual care" in practice may not be so much about caring for a spirit as it is about a way of being in practice.

Barnum (1996) suggested several "general methods" for nurses providing spiritual care including prayer and facilitating access to religious counselors and religious rites. Barnum also identified "patient-managed therapies" suggesting that "faith is an important spiritual therapy for patients" and concluded that "whether the spiritual therapies for patients are self-applied or administered by the nurse, much of the literature treats spiritual therapies as tactics to relieve stress" (p. 159). Barnum's concern seems to be the delineation and differentiation of spiritual therapies as distinct from other therapies such as psychological. What is not at all questioned, however, is the notion that faith can be "applied" as a "therapy." Here again, the influence of the natural sciences is seen in the view that faith is a thing, an object that can be manipulated like other objects.

Similar ideas are implied in the stated purpose of another study (Taylor, Amenta, & Highfield, 1995), "to determine what spiritual care practices oncology nurses use," suggesting a technology rather than a way of being (Bishop & Scudder, 1995). The findings of this study indicated that nurses consider spiritual care practices to include praying with patients, referring to chaplains or clergy, and providing religious materials. However, nurses also identified that "spiritual care" included serving as a therapeutic presence, listening, and talking to patients. Other studies of both nurses and patients have reported similar findings, reporting both "doing" and "being" practices as important for spiritual care (Bauer & Barron, 1995; Hall & Lanig, 1993; Taylor et al., 1995; Reed, 1992; Tuck, Pullen, & Lynn, 1997; Tuck et al., 2001).

Only two studies (Stiles, 1990; Wright et al., 1996) were identified that examined spirituality in relation to families. Both identified the embedded nature of spirituality in nursing practices in the nursing of families and in family systems nursing.

Using an ethnographic approach, Stiles (1990) explored the nature of the nurse-family spiritual relationship using an open-ended interview process with 11 hospice nurses and 12 families in bereavement. The guiding question, "What was your hospice experience like?" avoided direct inquiry into spirituality because the researcher preferred to allow a spiritual dimension to emerge if it was salient to the participants. Five themes were identified that reflected spiritual experiences in the relationship. These include:

1. Ways of being with (for example, being available, sharing, listening, humor)
2. Ways of doing (physical care, touch, explaining)
3. Ways of knowing (families drew on nurses'

> knowledge of the dying process and the transcendent)

4. Ways of receiving and giving (including mutual opportunities for growth)
5. Ways of welcoming a stranger (entrusting loved ones to the nurse, sharing the hospice experience)

Findings indicated that the "nurse-family relationship is mutual and dialogic and fosters growth for both nurses and families" (p. 235).

A second study (Wright et al., 1996), guided by hermeneutics, explored nursing interventions with families having difficulties living with a range of serious illnesses. Although the focus of the study was not specifically about spirituality, in therapeutic conversations with the families the authors found that "a discourse of suffering frequently opens up a discourse of spirituality" (p. 63). This study points to the need to understand more about how it is that a discourse of spirituality is opened up and is kept open and what difference this makes to families.

Although not a formal inquiry, in a clinical case analysis of the ways in which family systems nurses open space to spirituality, four practices were identified (McLeod & Wright, 2001). These included (1) opening space for the gift of listening, (2) maintaining curiosity and openness to surprise, (3) inviting reflection on spiritual/religious beliefs, and (4) the invocation of metaphor. Practices were embedded in the therapeutic conversations that evolved among the nurse, the family, and the clinical team.

SPIRITUAL PREFERENCES

In addition to the literature exploring spirituality in health and illness, there are survey findings and studies of patients' preferences, suggesting that health professionals should be aware of, and attend to, spirituality to a greater extent than they do now. For example, survey findings in Canada highlight the importance of religious and spiritual beliefs of Canadians. According to the *MacLean*'s magazine religion poll (Chisholm & Steele, 1993), approximately 75 percent of the population profess Christian beliefs and an association with a Christian denomination. In addition, between 77 and 90 percent profess a belief in God (depending on the region of the country) and identify with particular faiths or denominations and between 68 and 83 percent believe that God "cares about me" personally (Bibby, 2002).

In relation to health-care practices, surveys in the United States have identified that up to 40 percent of individuals would consider it very important for their physician to address spiritual issues with them if they were seriously ill (Gallup, 1997), and 77 percent of inpatients in another study wanted their physicians or counselors to address their spiritual needs (King & Bushwick, 1994). Moadel and colleagues (1999), in a sample of 248 ethnically diverse people living with cancer, identified a variety of spiritual and existential needs. Patients indicated they wanted help from health professionals with overcoming their fears (51%), finding hope (42%), finding meaning in life (28%), finding spiritual resources

(39%), or having someone to talk with about finding peace of mind (43%), the meaning of life (28%), and dying and death (25%).

In another Gallup poll (1996), 66 percent of respondents stated that, in a counseling situation, they would prefer that their caregivers represent spiritual values and beliefs, and more than 81 percent would prefer a caregiver who enabled them to integrate their values and belief system into the counseling process. Griffith (1995) reported that clients "want to reflect on spiritual experiences in therapy, and...feel fragmented by attempting to delegate psychological, relational issues to conversations with their therapist and spiritual issues to conversations with their priest, rabbi, or pastor" (p. 124). These findings provide some indication of how important spirituality might be to persons experiencing serious illness and the need for health professionals to attend to these concerns.

Within the nursing literature, there are mixed findings about how well nurses meet these needs. Some suggest that nurses can and do understand and provide what might be considered good spiritual care (Eifried, 1998; Stiles, 1990; Wright et al., 1996), whereas others suggest that there are significant limitations in nurses' understanding and in their willingness to provide spiritual care (Hall & Lanig, 1993; Highfield & Cason, 1983; Kristeller et al., 1999; Tuck et al., 1997).

From this review of the literature about spiritual care practices, it appears that the way in which the questions are asked, the educational level and age of study participants, and the practice setting influence the findings. What seems to vary is the participants' ability to articulate this aspect of their practice, depending on how the question is framed and the aforementioned demographic variables. Even if nurses may feel uncertain about spiritual care when asked (Kristeller et al., 1999; Emblen, 1992; Emblen & Pesut, 2001; Taylor et al., 1995; Tuck et al., 1997), this does not mean that nurses are not providing spiritual care.

Rather, nurses provide spiritual care that is embedded in other caring practices and therefore is less visible and more tacit. Helping to make visible the tacit through studies of lived experience in practice may contribute to nurses' ability to articulate and ultimately strengthen spiritual care practices.

Tensions and Future Directions

There are two primary and related tensions in the literature that influence the future directions: the struggle with language and the implications of the objectification of spirituality for nursing practice.

The Struggle with Language

The first struggle is the language of spirituality and religion. There is clearly a need to delineate between these two concepts, but language that is too definitive is also problematic. The objectifying language of the natural sciences sometimes suggests that nurses can care for a "spirit" as if it were a thing that we could hold in our hands.

Such methodic knowledge of spirituality does not make it easier to understand spirituality in practice. Instead, objectification makes spirituality less recognizable because spirituality always embodies a struggle in reaching beyond that which is human to that which transcends our humanness. Understanding spirituality in practice requires that we live with the fact that as it emerges in practice, it *is* ambiguous and multivocal, particular and local.

Rather than supporting nursing practice in its attention to the spiritual domain, such knowledge may be more alienating. Simplifying what is necessarily complex for the sake of procedural knowledge results in simplified interventions that may be less useful. However, there is value contained in the struggle to describe, or to bring into language, a lived experience of spirituality, as long as that struggle does not drift toward a terminal meaning.

The Objectification of Spirituality

The development of "interventions" follows from the identification of "spiritual needs," with both reflecting, at least to an extent, the objectification of spirituality as something that can be assessed and treated. This, of course, raises many questions, some of which have already been alluded to. For example, do we, as nurses, believe that spirituality can be "assessed" in this way? Do we believe that questions of spirituality can be asked, answered, and recorded in the same way as we record fluid intake (Mayer, 1992)? That we "intervene" with spiritual problems? What do such beliefs imply about our relationships with clients and with the sacred? What implications do they have for nurses, who are exhorted to assess and intervene? Is it even reasonable to expect that most nurses will be able to "intervene" well?

What is clear from the review of theory and research is that there are at least two fairly distinct voices about spiritual care practices that reflect certain epistemological assumptions and that have implications for nursing practice. The quieter voice is articulating the lived experience of spirituality. Few of these studies, however, have explored spirituality as a practice in nursing care generally or family nursing specifically.

Far more prominent in the literature is the voice that, congruent with the natural science traditions, understands spirituality as an object, one that can be assessed, measured, quantified, and with which a nurse "intervenes." This standpoint is consistent with the literature in other disciplines investigating spirituality (religion) and health (Ellison & Levin, 1998; Koenig et al., 2001). Such an approach may be useful from an epidemiological perspective in validating the importance of spirituality and religion to health and illness. It is more difficult, however, to imagine how one will develop "interventions" based on the body of literature that will emerge from a research agenda informed by these understandings. Can Koenig and colleagues (2001) be serious when they suggest, in their section on future directions for research, that "research is needed to determine what types of religious coping are effective for what types of life stress" (p. 468) so that interventions can be designed? Are religious belief and practice just other things that we manipulate as health-care practitioners?

Some (Emblen, 1992; Mayer, 1992) make the assumption that if spirituality and religion were more clearly defined, better nursing practice would be the result. However, if spirituality in nursing practice is largely tacit, embodied in care, clear definition will not contribute to the kind of understanding needed but rather result in some rather bizarre recommendations.

For example, Carson (1989) suggested that appropriate goals for nursing intervention in the case of spiritual distress include promoting clients' spiritual beliefs and promoting or maintaining clients' relationships with their personal deity. Outcomes that might be expected from good spiritual care include that patients will express decreased feelings of guilt and anxiety, religious or spiritual satisfaction, being at peace, and positive meanings about their existence and present circumstances, while displaying positive affect and behavior. No less daunting is the message of Simsen (1988) that a patient's ability to find meaning in his or her illness depends on the skills of knowing, hoping, and trusting and that these skills can be taught by nurses as a central part of spiritual care.

It is little wonder that some nurses are uncomfortable with spiritual care and perhaps see it as an impossible task when it is defined in these ways. There are more questions that arise out of such descriptions of spiritual care. Is it realistic to think that nurses can promote or maintain someone else's relationship with a personal deity or be responsible for another finding meaning in their life circumstances? What kind of knowledge is needed to do this? What do such goals imply about the nature of the nurse-patient relationship?

Nurses make choices about the ways in which they position themselves in relation to patients and families. Such choices have implications for these relationships. Drawing on the philosopher Emmanuel Levinas, Frank (1998) suggested, "There is an inextricable relation between knowing the other, being known by the other and knowing oneself. When this relation is forgotten, attention ceases to be a gift and becomes reduced to instrumental necessity" (p. 200).

In the objectification of spirituality, which leads to "assessment" and "intervention," this relation *is* forgotten. It is also a positioning that invites a view of the nurse as one who is the expert rather than a participant in the struggle to live with illness. The relationship becomes one of hierarchy, of "acting" on, potentially one of manipulation, rather than one of respectful "being with." The nurse is the one who "intervenes," "promotes," and "maintains." The nurse's limitations in this area are rarely acknowledged except to say that nurses are "uncomfortable" with spiritual care because of lack of clarity in definition (Emblen, 1992; Mayer, 1992), lack of education (Narayansamy, 1993), or role confusion (Fry, 1998).

Although nurses have an obligation to become experienced, even wise, about spirituality, no general intervention will suffice. What might suffice instead would be to consider care generally, and spiritual care specifically, as a dialogic, hermeneutic process, "not an aggregate of anonymous truths, but a human comportment" (Gadamer, 1999, p. 18).

Future Directions

There is clearly a need to understand more about the meaning of spirituality in nursing practice as it is lived. Nurses continually address (and are addressed by) concerns and questions that can be considered spiritual and/or religious and need to become experienced in good conduct in the face of such questions. In addition, although most definitions and conceptualizations of spirituality include acknowledgment of the spiritual nature of relationships, and the communal aspect of spirituality, only one study (Stiles, 1990) was identified that explicitly explored spirituality from a nurse-family perspective. This would seem to be a significant gap, limiting practice development in the area of family nursing.

Within the family nursing community, there has been a clarion call for a greater focus on nursing interventions and outcomes in family research (Gilliss & Knafl, 1999; Wright & Bell, 1994). There is considerable descriptive research about families' experiences of illness but little research that points to how nurses might conduct themselves well with regard to spirituality. There is certainly a need to know if nurses have helped a family, as well as a need to make sense out of what helped by looking inside interventions (Wright & Bell, 1994).

References

Adams, N. (1995). Spirituality, science and therapy. *Australian and New Zealand Journal of Family Therapy, 16*(4), 201–208.

Anderson, D.A., & Worthen, D. (1997). Exploring a fourth dimension: Spirituality as a resource for the couple therapist. *Journal of Marital and Family Therapy, 23*(1), 3–12.

Anderson, H. (1999). Feet planted firmly in midair: A spirituality for family living. In F. Walsh (Ed.), *Spiritual resources in family therapy* (pp. 157–176). New York: Guilford.

Anderson, H., & Goolishian, H.A. (1988). Human systems as linguistic systems: Preliminary and evolving ideas about the implications for clinical theory. *Family Process, 27*(4), 371–393.

Ballard, A., Green, T., McCaa, A., & Logsdon, M.C. (1997). A comparison of the level of hope in patients with newly diagnosed and recurrent cancer. *Oncology Nursing Forum, 24*(5), 899–904.

Barnhart, R.K. (Ed.). (1988). *The Barnhart dictionary of etymology.* New York: H.W. Wilson.

Barnum, B.S. (1996). *Spirituality in nursing: From traditional to new age.* New York: Springer.

Bauer, T., & Barron, C.R. (1995). Nursing interventions for spiritual care. Preferences of the community based elderly. *Journal of Holistic Nursing, 13*(3), 268–279.

Becvar, D. (1996). *Soul healing: A spiritual orientation to counseling and therapy.* New York: Basic Books.

Benson, H. (1996). *Timeless healing: The power and biology of belief.* New York: Fireside.

Bergin, A. (1991). Values and religious issues in psychotherapy and mental health. *American Psychologist, 4,* 394–403.

Bibby, R. (1987). *Fragmented Gods: The poverty and potential of religion in Canada.* Toronto: Irwin.

Bibby, R. (1993). *Unknown Gods: The ongoing story of religion in Canada.* Toronto: Stoddart.

Bibby, R. (2002). *Restless Gods: The renaissance of religion in Canada.* Toronto: Stoddard.

Bird, J. (2000). *The heart's narrative: Therapy and navigating life's contradictions.* Auckland, New Zealand: Edge.

Bishop, A.H., & Scudder, J.R., Jr. (1995). Applied science, practice, and intervention technology. In A. Omery, C.E. Kasper, & G.G. Page (Eds.), *In search of nursing science* (pp. 263–274). Thousand Oaks, CA: Sage.

Boyd-Franklin, N., & Lockwood, T.W. (1999). Spirituality and religion. Implications for psychotherapy with African American clients and families. In F. Walsh (Ed.), *Spiritual resources in family therapy* (pp .90–103). New York: Guilford.

Brittain, J. (1986). Theological foundations for spiritual care. *Journal of Religion and Health, 25*(2), 107–120.

Burkhardt, M.A. (1989). Spirituality: An analysis of the concept. *Holistic Nursing Practice, 3*(3), 69–77.

Burkhardt, M.A. (1994). Becoming and connecting: Elements of spirituality for women. *Holistic Nursing Practice, 8*(4), 12–21.

Burnard, P. (1987). Spiritual distress and the nursing response: Theoretical considerations and counseling skills. *Journal of Advanced Nursing, 12*, 377–382.

Capra, F., & Steindl-Rast, D. (1991). *Belonging to the universe: Explorations on the frontiers of science and spirituality.* San Francisco: Harper & Row.

Carlson, T.D., & Erickson, M.J. (2002). A conversation about spirituality in marriage and family therapy: Exploring the possibilities. *Journal of Family Psychotherapy, 13*(1/2), 1–12.

Carlson, T.D., Kirkpatrick, D., Hecker, L., & Killmer, M. (2002). Religion, spirituality, and marriage and family therapy: A study of family therapists' beliefs about the appropriateness of addressing religious and spiritual issues in therapy. *American Journal of Family Therapy, 30*, 157–171.

Carson, V. (1989). *Spiritual dimensions of nursing practice.* Philadelphia: Saunders.

Carter, B. (2000). The salvation of souls: But what is a soul? *Perspectives on Science and Christian Faith, 42*(4), 242–254.

Chisholm, P., & Steele, S. (1993). Sacred and profane: Living with Christianity in a secular world. Special report: The religion poll. *MacLean's, 106*(15), 40–43.

Chiu, L. (2000). Lived experience of spirituality in

Taiwanese women with breast cancer. *Western Journal of Nursing Research, 22*(1), 29–53.

Chubb, H., Gutsche, S., & Efron, D. (1994). Spirituality, religion, and world view. Introduction to the special issue. *Journal of Systemic Therapies, 13*(3), 1–6.

Clarke, C., Cross, J., Deane, D., & Lowry, L. (1991). Spirituality: Integral to quality care. *Holistic Nursing Practice, 5*(3), 67–76.

Cusveller, B. (1998). Cut from the right wood: Spiritual and ethical pluralism in professional nursing practice. *Journal of Advanced Nursing, 28*(2), 266–273.

Dossey, B.M., Keegan, L., Guzzetta, C.E., & Kolkmeier, L.G. (1995). *Holistic nursing: A handbook for practice* (2nd ed.). Gaithersburg, MD: Aspen.

Dossey, L. (1993). *Healing words: The power of prayer and the practice of medicine.* San Francisco: Harper.

Dyson, J., Cobb, M., & Forman, D. (1997). The meaning of spirituality: A literature review. *Journal of Advanced Nursing, 26,* 1183–1188.

Eifried, S. (1998). Helping patients find meaning: A caring response to suffering. *International Journal of Human Caring, 2*(1), 33–39.

Elkins, D.N. (1999). Spirituality. *Psychology Today, 32*(5), 44–48.

Ellison, C.G., & Levin, J.S. (1998). The religion-health connection: Evidence, theory, and future directions. *Health Education and Behavior, 25*(6), 700–720.

Emblen, J.D. (1992). Religion and spirituality de-fined according to current use in nursing litera-ture. *Journal of Professional Nursing, 8*(1), 41–47.

Emblen, J., & Halstead, L. (1993). Spiritual needs and interventions: Comparing views of patients, nurses, and chaplains. *Clinical Nurse Specialist, 7*(4), 175–182.

Emblen, J., & Pesut, B. (2001). Strengthening transcendental meaning: A model for the spiritual nursing care of patients experiencing suffering. *Journal of Holistic Nursing, 19*(1), 42–56.

Feher, S., & Maly, R.C. (1999). Coping with breast cancer in later life: The role of religious faith. *Psycho-Oncology, 8*(5), 408–416.

Fehring, R.J., Miller, J.F., & Shaw, C. (1997). Spiritual well-being, religiosity, hope, depression, and other mood states in elderly people coping with cancer. *Oncology Nursing Forum, 24*(4), 663–671.

Fernsler, J.I., Klemm, P., & Miller, M.A. (1999). Spiritual well-being and demands of illness in people with colorectal cancer. *Cancer Nursing, 22*(2), 134–140.

Ferrell, B.R., Grant, M., Funk, B., Garcia, N., Otis-Green, S., & Schaffner, M.L.J. (1996). Quality of life in breast cancer. *Cancer Practice, 4*(6), 331–340.

Frank, A.W. (1998). Just listening: Narrative and deep illness. *Families, Systems, & Health, 16*(6), 197–212.

Fredette, S.L. (1995). Breast cancer survivors: Concerns and coping. *Cancer Nursing, 18*(1), 35–46.

Fry, A. (1998). Spirituality, communication and mental health nursing: The tacit interdiction. *Australian and New Zealand Journal of Mental Health Nursing, 7*, 25–32.

Fryback, P.B., & Reinert, B.R. (1999). Spirituality and people with potentially fatal diagnoses. *Nursing Forum, 34*(1), 13–22.

Gadamer, H.G. (1999). *Hermeneutics, religion, & ethics*. (J. Weinsheimer, Trans.). New Haven, CT: Yale University Press.

Gallup, G., Jr. (1996). *Religion in America. 1996 report*. Princeton, NJ: Princeton Religion Research Centre.

Gallup, H. (1997). *Spiritual beliefs and the dying process. A report on a national survey*. Princeton, NJ: The George H. Gallup International Institute.

Gartner, J.D. (1996). Religious commitment, mental health, prosocial behavior: A review of the empirical literature. In E.P. Shafranske (Ed.), *Religion and the clinical practice of psychology*. Washington, DC: American Psychological Association.

Gilliss, C.L., & Knafl, K.A. (1999). Nursing care of families in non-normative transitions. In A.S. Hinshaw, S.L. Feetham, & J.L. Shaver (Eds.), *Handbook of clinical nursing research* (pp. 231–249). Thousand Oaks, CA: Sage.

Griffith, J.L., & Griffith, M.E. (2002). *Encountering the sacred in psychotherapy: How to talk with people about their spiritual lives*. New York: The Guilford Press.

Griffith, M.E. (1995). Opening therapy to conversations with a personal God. *Journal of Feminist Family Therapy, 7*(1/2), 123–139.

Hall, C. & Lanig, H. (1993). Spiritual caring behaviors as reported by Christian nurses. *Western Journal of Nursing Research, 15*(6), 730–741.

Hermann, C.P. (2001). Spiritual needs of dying patients: A qualitative study. *Oncology Nursing Forum, 28*(1), 67–72.

Highfield, M., & Cason, C. (1983). Spiritual needs of patients: Are they recognized? *Cancer Nursing, 6*(3), 187–192.

Hoffman, L. (1990). Constructing realities: An art of lenses. *Family Process, 29,* 1–12.

Imber-Black, E., Roberts, J., & Whiting, R. (Eds.). (1993). *Rituals in families and family therapy.* New York: W. W. Norton.

Joanides, C. (1997). A qualitative investigation of the meaning of religion and spirituality to a group of Orthodox Christians: Implications for marriage and family therapy. *Journal of Family Social Work, 2*(4), 59–76.

Keegan, L. (1994). *The nurse as healer.* New York: Delmar.

Kim, M.J., McFarland, G.K., & McLane, A.M. (1987). *Pocket guide to nursing diagnosis* (2nd ed.). St. Louis: C.V. Mosby.

King, D.E., & Bushwick, B. (1994). Beliefs and attitudes of hospital inpatients about faith healing and prayer. *Journal of Family Practice, 39,* 349–352.

Koenig, H.G. (1995). *Research in religion and aging.* Westport, CT: Greenwood.

Koenig, H.G., McCullough, M.E., & Larson, D.B. (2001). *Handbook of religion and health.* New York: Oxford University.

Kristeller, J.L., Zumbrun, C.S., & Schilling, R.F. (1999). 'I would if I could': How oncologists and oncology nurses address spiritual distress in cancer patients. *Psycho-Oncology, 8*(5), 451–458.

Kurtz, M.E., Wyatt, G., & Kurtz, J.C. (1995). Psychological and sexual well-being, philosophical/spiritual views, and health habits of long-term cancer survivors. *Health Care for Women International, 16*(3), 253–262.

Larson, D.B. (1993). *The faith factor: An annotated bibliography of systematic reviews and clinical research on spiritual subjects.* (Vol. 2). Radnor, PA: John Templeton Foundation.

Larson, D.B. (2001, May). *Spirituality and Health: What does the research say?* Paper presented at the North American Multidisciplinary Conference on Spirituality and Health, Calgary, AB.

Laukhuf, G., & Werner, H. (1998). Spirituality: The missing link. *Journal of Neuroscience Nursing, 30*(1), 60–67.

Lukoff, D., Lu, F., & Turner, R. (1992). Toward a more culturally sensitive DSM-IV. *The Journal of Nervous Disease, 180*(11), 673–682.

Marshall, E.S., Olsen, S.F., Mandleco, B.L., Dyches, T.T., Allred, K.W., & Sansom, N. (2003). "This is a spiritual experience": Perspectives of Latter-Day Saint Families living with a child with disabilities. *Qualitative Health Research, 13*(1), 57–76.

Martsolf, D.S., & Mickley, J.R. (1998). The concept of spirituality in nursing theories: Differing world views and extent of focus. *Journal of Advanced Nursing, 27,* 294–303.

Mathews, D.A., Larson, D.B., & Barry, C.P. (1993). *The faith factor: An annotated bibliography of systematic reviews and clinical research on spiritual subjects.* (Vol. 1). Radnor, PA: John Templeton Foundation.

Mayer, J. (1992). Wholly responsible for a part, or partly responsible for a whole? *Second Opinion, 17*(3), 26–55.

McLeod, D.L., & Wright, L.M. (2001). Conversations of spirituality: Spirituality in family systems nursing—Making the case with four clinical vignettes. *Journal of Family Nursing, 7*(4), 391–415.

McSherry, W., & Draper, P. (1998). The debates emerging from the literature surrounding the concept of spirituality as applied to nursing. *Journal of Advanced Nursing, 27,* 683–691.

Mickley, J.R., Carson, V., & Soeken, K.L. (1995). Religion and adult mental health: State of the science in nursing. *Issues in Mental Health Nursing, 16,* 345–360.

Moadel, A., Morgan, C., Fatone, A., Grennan, J., Carter, J., Laruffa, G., et al. (1999). Seeking meaning and hope: Self-reported spiritual and existential needs among an ethnically diverse cancer patient population. *Psycho-Oncology, 8*(5), 378–385.

Moore, T. (1992/1994). *Care of the soul.* New York: Harper Collins.

Moore, T. (1994). *Soul mates.* New York: Harper Collins.

Mytko, J.L., & Knight, S.J. (1999). Body, mind and spirit: Towards the integration of religiosity and spirituality in cancer quality of life research. *Psycho-Oncology, 8*(5), 439–450.

Nagai-Jacobson, M.G. & Burkhardt, M.A. (1989). Spirituality: Cornerstone of holistic nursing practice. *Holistic Nursing Practice, 3*(3), 18–26.

Narayansamy, A. (1993). Nurses' awareness and educational preparation in meeting their patients' spiritual needs. *Nurse Education Today, 13,* 196–201.

Nelson, S. (2000). *A genealogy of care of the sick: Nursing, holism and pious practice.* Southsea, Great Britain: Nursing Praxis International.

Neuman, B. (1995). *The Neuman systems model* (3rd ed.). Norwalk, CT: Appleton & Lange.

Newman, M.A. (1994). *Health as expanding consciousness* (2nd ed.). New York: National League for Nursing.

Nightingale, F. (1859/1969). *Notes on nursing: What it is and what it is not.* New York: Dover.

O'Brien, M.E. (1999). *Spirituality in nursing: Standing on holy ground.* Sudberry, MA: Jones & Bartlett.

Oldnall, A.S. (1995). On the absence of spirituality in nursing theories and models. *Journal of Advanced Nursing, 21*, 417–418.

Prest, L.A., & Keller, J.F. (1993). Spirituality and family therapy: Spiritual beliefs, myths, and metaphors. *Journal of Marital and Family Therapy, 19*(2), 137–148.

Reed, P.G. (1992). An emerging paradigm for the investigation of spirituality in nursing. *Research in Nursing and Health, 15*, 349–357.

Richards, P.S., & Bergin, A.E. (1997). *A spiritual strategy for counseling and psychotherapy.* Washington, DC: American Psychological Association.

Simsen, B. (1988). Nursing the spirit. *Nursing Times, 84*(37), 31–33.

Smucker, C. (1996). A phenomenological description of the experience of spiritual distress. *Nursing Diagnosis, 7*(2), 81–91.

Stewart, S.P., & Gale, J.E. (1994). On hallowed ground: Marital therapy with couples on the religious right. *Journal of Systemic Therapies, 13*(3), 16–25.

Stiles, M.K. (1990). The shining stranger: Nurse-family spiritual relationship. *Cancer Nursing, 13*(4), 235–245.

Stoll, R.I. (1979). Guidelines for spiritual assessment. *American Journal of Nursing, 79*, 1574–1577.

Swenson, D.S. (1999*). Society, spirituality and the sacred. A social scientific introduction.* Peterborough, Ontario: Broadview.

Tanyi, R.A. (2002). Towards clarification of the meaning of spirituality. *Journal of Advanced Nursing, 39*(5), 500–509.

Taylor, P.B., Amenta, M., & Highfield, M. (1995).

Spiritual care practices of oncology nurses. *Oncology Nursing Forum, 22*, 31–39.

Tuck, I., Pullen, L., & Lynn, C. (1997). Spiritual interventions provided by mental health nurses. *Western Journal of Nursing Research, 19*(3), 351–363.

Tuck, I., Pullen, L., & Wallace, D. (2001). A comparative study of the spiritual perspectives and interventions of mental health and parish nurses. *Issues in Mental Health Nursing, 22*, 593–605.

Walsh, F. (1999). Overview. In F. Walsh, (Ed.), *Spiritual resources in family therapy* (pp. 3–27). New York: Guilford.

Walton, J. (1999). Spirituality of patients recovering from an acute myocardial infarction. A grounded theory study. *Journal of Holistic Nursing, 17*(1), 34–53.

Watson, J. (1988). *Nursing: Human science and human care.* Norwalk, CT: Appleton-Century Crofts.

Weaver, A.J., Flannelly, L.T., Flannelly, K.J., Koenig, H.G., & Larson, D.B. (1998). An analysis of research on religious and spiritual variables in three major mental health nursing journals. 1991–1995. *Issues in Mental Health Nursing, 19*, 263–276.

White C., & Tapping, C. (1990). Social justice and family therapy. *Dulwich Centre Newsletter, 1*, 1–46.

Widerquist, J. (1992). The spirituality of Florence Nightingale. *Nursing Research, 41*(1), 49–53.

Wright, L.M. (1999). Spirituality, suffering and beliefs: The soul of healing with families. In F. Walsh (Ed.), *Spiritual resources in families and family therapy* (pp. 61–75). New York: Guilford.

Wright, L.M., & Bell, J.M. (1994). The future of family nursing research: Interventions, interventions, interventions. *The Japanese Journal of Nursing Research, 27*(2–3), 4–15.

Wright, L.M., Watson, W.L., & Bell, J.M. (1996). *Beliefs: The heart of healing in families and illness*. New York: Basic Books.

Wyatt, G., & Friedman, L.L. (1996). Long-term female cancer survivors: Quality of life issues and clinical implications. *Cancer Nursing, 19*(1), 1–7.

4

The Trinity Model: Beliefs, Suffering, and Spirituality

Do we really need yet another model for nursing and nursing practice? It is my belief that models can be and are very useful for nurses and their practice. Models are helpful ways to bring collections of ideas, concepts, and notions into our awareness. Without this awareness, our nursing practice can appear to be haphazard and not based on any useful or organized thinking.

Therefore, I offer a new model, the Trinity Model, with the hope that it will provide nurses and other health-care professionals with a useful framework for thinking about the complex notions of beliefs, suffering, and spirituality. This is an overarching model for practice. However, models cannot stand alone. They are built on a foundation of many world views, theories, premises, and assumptions that inform the models that arise. Models in nursing practice are more understandable and meaningful if the underlying theories are articulated and made known. Therefore, to comprehend and use the Trinity Model in nursing practice with individuals and families, it is important to know the theoretical assumptions underlying this model. Underlying theoretical assumptions of any model are important to state because they are the foundation of the way in which those models are operationalized. The three theoretical foundations and world views that inform the Trinity Model are postmodernism (Kermode & Brown, 1996; Moules, 2000;

Tapp & Wright, 1996; Watson, 1995), systems theory (von Bertalanffy, 1974), and a biology of cognition (Maturana & Varela, 1992). These three theoretical foundations can be read about in more depth by the original authors or in a condensed manner in Wright and Leahey's (2000) Third Edition of *Nurses and Families: A Guide to Family Assessment and Intervention* and Wright, Watson, and Bell's (1996) *Beliefs: The Heart of Healing in Families and Illness.*

During the past few years, I have come to realize that a new trinity has emerged in my nursing practice, namely, beliefs, suffering, and, spirituality. I have had the privilege of engaging in hundreds of therapeutic conversations about serious illness with individuals and family members. These conversations invariably include family members' descriptions of suffering, the meaning they give to their suffering from spiritual domains, and their beliefs about their illness experience. I have become a passionate observer of and participant in the healing effect and changes that occur in the biopsychosocial-spiritual structure of clients, family members, and myself.

I now find it impossible to talk or think about spirituality without thinking about suffering and beliefs. And I find it equally impossible to think about suffering without talking about spirituality and beliefs. These three concepts or notions are thoroughly intertwined and closely related. However, I initially discuss each of these concepts separately because language constricts us from talking about them simultaneously.

I conceptualize the Trinity Model as the interrelatedness and interconnection of the three concepts—beliefs, suffering, and spirituality. It is at the confluence or intersection of these three concepts that life meaning and purpose are queried, questioned, found, affirmed, or challenged (Fig. 4–1). All three of these concepts need to be inquired about, explored, and examined when caring for persons and families experiencing serious illness, disability, loss, or trauma.

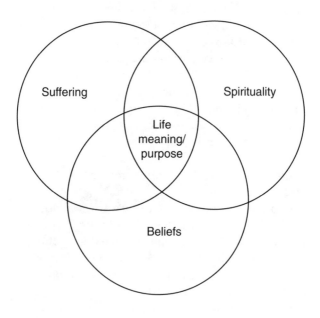

FIG. 4–1. The Trinity Model.

Beliefs in the Trinity Model

In our daily lives, the best medium for hearing our own and others' beliefs is the stories we exchange in our conversations. Beliefs are the blueprints from which we construct our lives and proceed to intermingle them with the lives of others (Wright et al, 1996). At no time are family and individual beliefs more affirmed, challenged, or threatened than when serious illness emerges. What one believes about illness contributes dramatically to how one experiences an illness. No two people and no two families have the same experience with the same disease, whether it is the common cold or multiple sclerosis. Some families view illness as a sign that they are sinful and disease as a punishment for ungodly living. Other families believe that being ill is a natural physical sign that the ill member should slow down and take care of himself or herself, that he or she can no longer neglect his or her health. There are also many beliefs about how family members should behave when illness enters a family.

Consequently, how families adapt, manage, and cope with illness arise from their beliefs about the illness that is confronting them. In fact, it may not be a particular illness that is a problem for a patient and his or her family, but rather the patient's and family's beliefs about the illness. Some individuals and family members cope very well with serious illness, but others do not; this is all related to their beliefs about the illness. What individuals and families believe about the illness, more than anything else, influences how they cope with the illness.

The beliefs of family members are often recon-structed after the experience of illness (that is, blueprints are revised); conversely, the beliefs of family members influence and shape the processes and outcomes of illness. For example, how family members treat even the common cold depends on their beliefs concerning how the person "caught" the cold in the first place. If one believes that colds are related to experi-ences of stress, one will probably treat the cold differently than if one believes a cold is caused by inadequate rest and working long hours. If one believes that the best remedy for a cold is to rest, drink plenty of fluid, and take vitamin C, that regimen will probably be followed.

If the treatment or remedy does not work, will the belief about the cause of the illness be main-tained? Will there be more openness to other treatment options when their original beliefs about the etiology and the cure of an illness have been challenged? Of course, there are cir-cumstances when beliefs may have little or no influence over the reaction of the body. Not all beliefs matter in the experience of an illness. It is the core beliefs that are most useful to un-cover and explore with families about their ill-ness experience: beliefs about the etiology/cause of illness, diagnosis of illness, healing and treatment, prognosis/outcome, mastery/control and influence on illness, the place of illness in our lives and relationships, the role of family members, the role of health-care professionals, and spirituality and religion in relation to illness (Wright et al, 1996).

Nurses bring their own strong personal and professional beliefs about illness to the patients, families, and clinical domain. Their beliefs influence how they view, assess, and, most important, care for and intervene with their patients and families. For example, nurses' beliefs about etiology may influence how a patient and family are received, perceived, and treated. A nurse who believes that obesity is a consequence of irresponsibility and personal weakness would be likely to respond differently to a family living with obesity than to a family living with the effects of a congenital heart defect, an illness over which a health professional may believe the individual or family has no control. The core beliefs of nurses that affect relationships with their patients and family members are their beliefs about illness, families, change, and their own role as nurses in the lives of their patients and families.

Some beliefs are more useful than others in coping with illness. To uncover the beliefs that are useful and those that are not, a simple dichotomy of beliefs can be useful: constraining beliefs versus facilitating beliefs (Wright et al., 1996). Family members hold beliefs about their problems that are constraining or facilitating. *Constraining beliefs* perpetuate problems and restrict options for alternative solutions to problems. *Facilitating beliefs* increase options for solutions to problems. Therefore, health professionals need to focus on identifying and challenging, altering, or modifying family members' constraining beliefs about illness and drawing forth, offering, and solidifying more facilitating beliefs. The outcome is, we hope, that the family experiences a new or renewed appreciation of their strengths and resources and increased options to discover and uncover solutions to their suffering. In the process, our beliefs as clinicians are continuously altered and modified from our involvement with patients and families.

My colleagues, Drs. Wendy Watson and Janice Bell, and I have substantially expanded on and embellished these ideas about beliefs, illness, and families in another text, *Beliefs: The Heart of Healing in Families and Illness.* Therefore I have highlighted only some of the aspects of beliefs in the context of illness in this chapter. The most important aspect to understand for the Trinity Model is to conceptualize the *reciprocity* on interaction among beliefs, suffering, and spirituality.

CLINICAL PRACTICE EXAMPLE: "ARE YOU BEHIND IN YOUR LIFE?"

I offer a clinical example of how exploring the illness beliefs of a young man opened space for his suffering and ultimately for a discourse on spirituality concerning the meaning and purpose of his life in the face of the impending death of his wife. Doran, a 32-year-old married man, sought assistance from the Family Nursing Unit (FNU), University of Calgary, to help him cope with the impending loss of his wife to Lou Gehrig's disease (amyotrophic lateral sclerosis). At the time of our clinical work with Doran, his wife, Josanne, had been hospitalized for 1 year and was paralyzed and incapable of verbal speech. Doran approached the FNU when the anniversary date of his wife's hospitalization neared 1 year. He attended four sessions at the FNU, during which he told the story of the effect of his wife's illness on his life. The following excerpts are from the clinical interviews that I was privileged to have with this young man. (LMW indicates Dr. Lorraine M. Wright. The client's name and that of his wife were changed for reasons of confidentiality.)

Doran: I'm very, very depressed, Dr. Wright, you know, I'm really fighting a depression a lot.

LMW: Are you? How do you know you're depressed?

Doran: It's just that I don't feel good; I don't feel good most of the time. After our last meeting, I went and saw my family doctor.

LMW: Yes...?

Doran: Because of some major heart problems I'm having because of all the stress I'm under. And I went to see him in the afternoon 2 weeks ago, and he listened to my chest, and I took a breathing test, right?

LMW: Yes...and?

Doran: And he hooked me up to an EKG and he said everything seems to be okay. He said everything seems normal; he just feels what's happening to me, is my heart is, I'm under so much stress right now....

LMW: Right.

Doran: Smoking and drinking coffee and stress. He said I'm definitely experiencing, you know, symptoms related to that. And he read my EKG and said there's no evidence of anything abnormal, right?

LMW: Umm....

Doran: But I'm getting these palpitations every day and it's scary 'cause I'm just always scared I'm just going to (*makes a sound here, like dropping dead*), you know?

LMW: Are you?

Doran: I'm scared I'm going to die because of it, yeah!

LMW: Really?

Doran: Yeah!

LMW: When did you start having this idea?

Doran: Well, about, well, I've been having these palpitations in my heart since November.

LMW: Yes, so are you saying that this is the scariest thing that you think about these days?

Doran: Well, it's everything....

LMW: It is the thought of you dying or is it the thought of Josanne dying that is the scariest? Which is the scariest thought? Yourself or Josanne?

Doran: Um... . I don't know.

LMW: If you had to choose, which is the scarier thought, to think about yourself dying or think about Josanne dying?

Doran: That's a tough one, you know... . I guess it would be the thought of me dying, you know. Um, knowing when Josanne dies, I mean, it's going to be a relief, you know?

LMW: A relief for whom, for Josanne, or for yourself?

> **Doran:** For both of us. She won't be suffering any more. And I won't be suffering; neither will her mother; neither will anybody else that's got to go up there and see her like that, you know?

Comments about Therapeutic Conversation

From this exploration, I learned how Doran's wife's illness was causing him to suffer both physically and emotionally. He shared his belief that he was fighting depression and revealed that he sought out medical advice about his palpitations but that no physical abnormalities were found. Both the physician and Doran believed that his palpitations were related to his present stressful situation of the serious life-threatening illness of his wife.

But much more was gleaned when I chose to "speak the unspeakable" (Wright et al., 1996) and to explore Doran's beliefs about "Which is the scarier thought, to think about yourself dying or thinking about Josanne dying?" This question created an opportunity for Doran to offer his feelings about his wife's impending death. This type of conversation between Doran and me opened space for suffering to be acknowledged and heard. It was during this part of the therapeutic conversation that Doran used the word "suffering" for the first time by stating that "she won't be suffering any more. I won't be suffering... ." Now we had a connection between his beliefs and his suffering. But I suspected that this was only the surface of his suffering, and I decided to gently explore its depths.

LMW: I'm going to ask you what might seem like a really harsh, a hard question. I don't mean it to sound as harsh, okay, as it may, Doran, but do you ever wish that she would die?

Doran: Yep (no hesitation). Yep, I wish that a lot.

LMW: Yes, because how would it make your life different?

Doran: How would it make my life different? I could go on with my life; I wouldn't be stuck like I am right now... . I'm living a nightmare right now.

LMW: So the anticipation of Josanne dying and the worry about yourself dying because of these heart palpitations, you are saying to me you feel you can't get on with your life, so if you can't get on with your life, are you behind in your life? Or is your life on hold?

Doran: My life is on hold, right now. Actually, I feel like I'm behind in my life...yes, I'm behind in my life. You know, I feel like I have nothing to live for, you know. It's so hard, I don't know how long this whole mess is gong to carry on for, and I don't know how many more months I'm going to have to go through this. I'm considering that I may not be strong enough to make it through the duration of my wife's illness and having to be out there and visiting her every day and trying to live two lives. I can't go on like that, that's the problem, you know, I don't know if I have the strength to go on.

Comments about Therapeutic Conversation

The depth of this young man's suffering was now raw and exposed and has led me into a discourse of spirituality. He was questioning whether he could live through this suffering or succumb to it by not being "strong enough." These conversations of suffering are indeed most difficult for me as a clinician, but I enter into them because of my strong belief that if suffering is exposed, then possibilities for healing can arise. When suffering is submerged and not acknowledged, it festers like a wound that eats away at the very spirit of a person.

Once Doran shared that he could not get on with his life while his wife was still living, the opportunity was presented for me to offer the notion that perhaps he might even believe that he was "behind in his life." This metaphor seemed to fit perfectly for Doran because he repeated this phrase back to me. Now we were entering into the spiritual domain by discussing the meaning and purpose of his life that caused him to behave in particular ways in the world toward himself and others. Through this therapeutic conversation, I learned that there was spiritual suffering in addition to his emotional and physical suffering.

Because of Doran's frank admission that he had nothing to live for, I now had the ethical responsibility to ask about possible suicidal thoughts. So I proceeded.

LMW: Umm. Do you ever have thoughts of killing yourself?

Doran: Oh, yeah.

LMW: How often do you entertain those ideas?

Doran: Well, I never really entertained those thoughts till lately, and it seems to be more and more.

LMW: That those thoughts trouble you more?

Doran: Sort of, but I'm a Catholic and I don't believe in it, I've always been taught that if I take my life, I won't go to heaven, you know.

LMW: Ummm. So do you think that this strong belief of yours will help you to get in the way or stop those thoughts of killing yourself?

Doran: I hope so, yeah.

LMW: I think that's a very good belief to have, isn't it? When you're troubled, it helps you to not take your life. Is there anything else; are there any other beliefs that you have that you think will help you?

Doran: No.

Comments about Therapeutic Conversation

The exploration of possible suicidal intentions leads to an important disclosure of Doran's religious beliefs regarding suicide. I chose to highlight this facilitating belief as one way to challenge his constraining belief that there was nothing for him to live for. It was at this point that I decided to validate his sadness and suffering—not about his wife's illness, but rather about his own suffering and the fact that he did not feel entitled to life.

LMW: Do you have any idea what I think about you at this moment?

Doran: I don't know.

LMW: What would you guess I think about you?

Doran: You feel sorry for me or whatever.

LMW: I don't think I feel as much sorry for you as I feel sad for you. Can I tell you why I feel sad for you? Would you be interested?

Doran: Yeah.

LMW: Okay. The reason that I feel sad for you is because I see at this point that you don't feel entitled to living.

Doran: Well, I want to live, I mean what's the point of living, you know? I mean I have nothing to look forward to right now.

LMW: Ah, so maybe it's a bit different then, so maybe you feel entitled to living but it's trying to find a good, a good reason for living.

Doran: Yeah.

LMW: Because at the moment so much is focused on people dying. You are thinking about yourself perhaps dying, you are thinking about Josanne dying? Is that so?

Doran: I guess so.

LMW: Okay. Well, let me ask you a few questions around that. May I? Are you a person, then, who believes that you always have to be getting on with your life, or that you can never be behind in your life?

Doran: Yeah. Well, I've always been ahead in my life, but you know, compared to most other people that I know, I'm behind in my life... .

LMW: So, I'm trying to understand this; this is really important. If you were ahead in your life at one time, but now you feel you are behind in your life, do you think you're still a little ahead in terms of what you have accomplished in your life, or are you falling far behind in your life right now?

Doran: Yeah, I don't have the things, like my sister's a year older than me and she's got, you know, a lot going for her, and other people I know who are the same age as me have a hell of a lot more going for them than I do.

LMW: And a lot is going for them in what sense? What's the biggest difference between them and you?

Doran: Well, they have their marriages, they have their homes, and they have, you know, things like that? They've got really good jobs, and for the most part they have a very clear idea of what they want out of life, but in my case, you know, I just can't seem to get myself going.

LMW: Well, let me ask you, it sounds to me like one place where you are ahead in your life, that your friends are not, and your sister, is your sister married?

Doran: Yeah.

LMW: Yes, okay, one of the places that I see that it seems you are ahead in your life is that most young men your age have not had to face the anticipation of their spouse dying...they usually do that when they're much older... .

Doran: Yeah, a lot of these men haven't had to face that and they have really good jobs, they've got marriages, they've got a handle on what they want out of life.

LMW: Well, I'm wondering then, how is it that a young man like yourself, who is ahead of yourself in your life in one sense that you have to anticipate your spouse dying, way before most men do, but you are behind in your life in the sense of like you said, in terms of a job, being able to go forward with your marriage... . But I'm trying to understand, how is it that you, Doran, have been given these challenges in life? How do you make sense of that?

Doran: I don't make sense of it... .

Comments about Therapeutic Conversation

Suffering tends to beg for explanation, and the lack of understanding about our suffering seems to invite us to suffer more. In this clinical conversation with Doran, I was struck once again that the meaning (beliefs) we harbor in relation to our suffering can increase or decrease our anguish. Doran went on.

Doran: I don't know, I try to figure it out and I can't figure it out, I just say, part of me just, when I think about that, right, part of me says, maybe if I was, I don't know.

LMW: Well, say more to me about that.

Doran: I say, "Why me"?

LMW: Yes, "Why you"?

Doran: Why me? Why can't it happen to somebody else? Why does this have to happen to me?

LMW: And why do you think?

Doran: I don't know. I don't have the answer to that.

LMW: So you are sort of stuck in this question, "Why me?" and not getting a satisfactory answer?

Doran: Yeah.

LMW: And do you believe it's possible to get an answer to this question, or are some questions never answered?

Comments about Therapeutic Conversation

The frequent question of "Why me?" was now plaguing Doran's mind. But one client eloquently taught me by saying, "Why NOT me? Why should I be spared suffering when others are not?" This is, of course, a very facilitating belief for the "Why me?" question involved in suffering. And Doran had his own facilitating belief that was now brought forth in conversation to help deal with his suffering.

Doran: Well, I believe that God's going to take care of me, you know, take care of my situation for me, I have to believe that.

LMW: Okay, so you believe that God will take care of you. Well, I think that's a very good belief to have.

Doran: Yeah?

LMW: Yes, and do you think this kind of belief could make you suicide proof?

Doran: Yeah, it could.

Comments about Therapeutic Conversation

Now I linked back to his thoughts of his life having no meaning and spoke the unspeakable once again by asking if his beliefs could help to make him suicide proof. This "unexpected context" (Tomm, 1987) question is useful for bringing forth something that has been masked or lost. In this case, Doran was asked to bring forth his lost identity of being "suicide proof." I extended this

line of questioning to sustain and distinguish
more facilitating beliefs.

LMW: How else do you know that you are suicide
proof?

Doran: Well, I've got people that really care about
me that would be, that in spite of how things are,
you know, I know that my Mom and Dad would always have their door wide open to me, right. If I ever
had to go there… .

LMW: Yes.

Doran: And stay with them for a few days there.

LMW: That's a wonderful thing to know, isn't it? Do
you feel that's a wonderful thing to have that kind of
backup?

Doran: Yeah, very much.

LMW: Okay, what other things make you suicide
proof?

Doran: Well, I think the fact that I've spoken about it.

LMW: So the fact that you're even talking about it
with me right now… .

Doran: Yeah… .

LMW: Is evidence that you're suicide proof?

Doran: Yeah, I think so.

LMW: Okay, that's very good. Anything else that
makes you suicide proof?

Doran: I have things to live for, I have to believe that
there's a better life for me, you know?

LMW: So you believe that there's a better life! Well,
that would certainly make a person suicide proof!

Doran: And I guess another one is I'm getting help
from different sources. I can come in here and I'm
seeing a friend for coffee regularly and that helps,
too.

Comments about Therapeutic Conversation

In my four sessions with Doran, his emotional and spiritual suffering decreased dramatically as he brought forth more facilitating beliefs about his situation. Also, neither Doran nor I nor our clinical team were worried any longer about possible suicide because he continued to believe that his life had meaning and purpose in the moment as well as in the future. Doran also began volunteering at the hospital where his wife was a patient, which was a truly selfless way to give more meaning to his life. This was a young man who was indeed "ahead in his life" in several domains. This clinical example exemplifies how our beliefs can invite suffering and ultimately lead to questions of spirituality.

Suffering in the Trinity Model

The alleviation of suffering has always been the heart of nursing. I believe that the ethical and obligatory goals of health-care professionals, especially nurses, must be to reduce, diminish, or alleviate (and, I hope, heal) emotional, physical, and/or spiritual suffering of patients and their family members. All forms of caring aim, in one way or another, to alleviate suffering (Lindholm & Eriksson, 1993). But what is suffering? Much has been written about suffering in a variety of disciplines, including nursing (Frank, 1994; Morse & Johnson, 1991). At the moment, my preferred way of conceptualizing or defining suffering is physical, emotional, or spiritual anguish, pain, or distress. Experiences of suffering can include serious illness that alters one's life and relationships as one knew them; the forced exclusion from everyday life; the strain of trying to endure; longing to love or be loved; acute or chronic pain; and conflict, anguish, or interference with love in relationships.

In a study by Hinds (1992), the suffering of family caregivers of noninstitutionalized cancer patients revealed descriptions such as fear of loneliness, uncertainty about the future, communication breakdown, and lack of support. Although I concur with these efforts to define and describe suffering, I most readily empathize with a patient who once described his suffering to me as "just feeling awful, preoccupied, and heavy most of the time."

Individual beliefs of patients and family members are involved in both the experience of suffering and making inferences from suffering. Certain beliefs may conserve or maintain an illness; others may exacerbate symptoms; others alleviate or diminish suffering (Wright et al., 1996). Suffering begs for an explanation of why it has occurred and how it can be endured! Through the exploration of beliefs with patients and families, it is possible to understand how they are attempting to have an explanation of why they are suffering. When nurses can invite persons to reflect on their beliefs, those persons often become more open to consider other possibilities.

Frank (1995) offers the idea that when persons turn their diseases into stories, they find healing. Listening to stories of illness is frequently more about listening to stories of suffering. From my clinical practice and research with families, I have come to strongly believe that talking about one's experience with illness can often alleviate or diminish emotional, physical, and/or spiritual suffering (Wright et al., 1996). To me, this talking about, witnessing, and listening to illness stories in therapeutic conversations become the context from which suffering can first be acknowledged and then alleviated when healing begins. And telling stories of illness invites the possibility of making sense of suffering. In short, talking is healing! (See Chapter 2 for further reflections about suffering.)

Spirituality in the Trinity Model

The influence of family members' spiritual and religious beliefs on their illness experiences has been one of the most neglected areas in individual and family nursing practice. However, there is much evidence that nurses are waking up to this neglected aspect of spirituality in human experience. Increasing numbers of articles have appeared in professional journals; several books are now available by nurses addressing this topic; and nursing and other health-care conferences have more presenters offering their ideas about spirituality. This is an encouraging and needed development in the health-care professions. (See Chapter 3 for a more indepth review of spirituality in the professional literature.)

My clinical experience with individuals and families has taught me that the experience of suffering from illness becomes transposed to one of spirituality as family members try to make meaning out of their suffering and distress. To understand how family members offer compassion and what efforts are made to alleviate suffering, it is imperative that nurses explore religious and spiritual beliefs in clinical work with families. It is through the medium of therapeutic conversations about the individual's and family members' experience with illness and their beliefs about the illness experience that a way of understanding, explaining, conversing, and creating changes and healing with our clients becomes visible.

The most significant learning about suffering that I have gained in my clinical work with individuals and families over 30 years is that a discourse on suffering invariably opens up a discourse on spirituality if families and nurses are open to it. Suffering invites and leads us into the spiritual domain. A shift to and emphasis on spirituality are frequently the most profound responses to suffering from illness. If nurses are to be helpful, we must acknowledge that suffering and often the senselessness of it are ultimately spiritual issues (Patterson, 1994). Spiritual distress may be experienced by an ill person or family member who is questioning the reason for her or his suffering.

A recent study offers credence to the very useful and helpful role that spirituality and spiritual beliefs can play right until the very end of life. Spirituality protects us against end-of-life despair, depression, and hopelessness. Researchers from Fordham University, Drs McLain, Rosenfeld, and Breitbart (2003), determined that no matter what their religion, terminally ill people who had been given less than 3 months to live but who had a sense of spiritual well-being were less likely to spend those last months in a state of despair. They were also less likely than nonspiritual people to feel hopeless, to want to die, or to consider suicide.

Previous research has shown repeatedly that spirituality can greatly ease the mental and emotional anguish that accompanies a host of medical ailments or the loss of a loved one. In the study by McLain and associates (2003) that involved interviews with 160 terminally ill people, spirituality was measured in two ways: inner peace and the comfort and strength they got from their religious faith. When someone is terminally ill, it is quite common and understandable to feel despair in the final days of life. But even when patients were depressed, they tended to want to die only if they had a low sense of spiritual well-being. Spiritual people who were depressed by their illness did not wish for a hastened death. "Spiritual well-being is a really crucial, central aspect of how you cope with death," study author Dr. Barry Rosenfeld of Fordham University in New York told *Reuters*.

My preferred way to conceptualize or define spirituality is as whatever or whoever gives ultimate meaning and purpose in one's life, which invites particular ways of being in the world in relation to others, oneself, and the universe.

CLINICAL PRACTICE EXAMPLE: "WHERE WILL I GO AFTER I DIE?"

The proof is always in the pudding! I offer the following clinical practice example to illuminate the interrelatedness and thus the trinity of beliefs, suffering, and spirituality.

This family consists of a 63-year-old man, Aaron; his 62-year-old wife, Miriam; and their two grown children, who live in a different city. Aaron had experienced a myocardial infarction 6 months before this session. The family had been seen for two sessions in an outpatient nursing clinic before I was invited for a consultation. The couple had made good progress in their two sessions with the Master's nursing student and reported to me that talking about how the illness had affected their marriage and had helped to bring forth a lot of worries and fears that both were experiencing. Consequently, the couple reported that they were now talking more at home, having breakfast together for the first time in many years, and feeling more understood by each other.

When I work with families in which one spouse has experienced a heart attack, I routinely ask the nonaffected partners if they worry about their spouses having another heart attack. I routinely do this because I have learned that this is one of the most common fears of the spouse of a heart attack survivor. It was also the case with this couple and proved to be a critical exploration that opened up even more alarming concerns. In this case, Miriam responded, "Yes, all the time." When I asked Aaron if he worried about having another heart attack, he confirmed that he *does not worry* about dying from another heart attack. The most fascinating aspect of this therapeutic inquiry occurred when Miriam disclosed her belief that *she* is going to have a heart attack! She also disclosed that she has been on antidepressant medication for 20 years because of her fear of dying. In the following verbatim transcript of my clinical work with this family, a significant distinction is made. (LMW indicates Dr. Lorraine M. Wright. The names of the husband and wife have been change for reasons of confidentiality.)

LMW: So when you say (*addresses Miriam*) that you have a fear of dying, what do you mean by that?

Miriam: I don't know where I'm going to go, that's the fear. I'm afraid. I don't know where I'm going to go, I don't know why. I mean I don't know if it's the religion, or the school, I mean it's the way I was brought up.

LMW: So, you're saying that the biggest worry around for you is not HOW you're going to die, is it? But where you're going to go AFTER you die?

Miriam: Exactly.

LMW: I see.

Miram: Exactly.

Comments about Therapeutic Conversation

This was a captivating and most important distinction and self-disclosure by this incredibly fearful woman. This dear woman clarified that it was not the fear of dying that was most troublesome, but rather her fear of where she was going to go *after* she dies. Further clarification of her beliefs then ensued.

Miriam: If you're good, then you're going to heaven, and if you're bad, you're going to hell. So it was always on my mind, everything was a sin, so I grew up like that and I was afraid of everything, and it's still on my mind today!

LMW: Hmmmm.

Miriam: So to me, I always see the clock (*gestures indicating a pendulum*) and if you're good (*gestures to one side*) and if you're bad (*gestures to the other side*) and there's no middle. I don't know where I'm going to go.

LMW: So when you evaluate our life today, Miriam, would you say... ?

Miriam: Well, I was bad sometimes, like everybody else... .

LMW: Sure... .

Miriam: But then many times or most of the times, but uh....

LMW: But when you evaluate your life now and you look at your life, do you feel good about how you've lived your life?

Miriam: Yes, sure... .

LMW: Do you think, uh... .

Miriam: Sure, I wouldn't change my life, even though we went through a lot, I mean, with family and everything, but I wouldn't change my life anyway.

LMW: I wonder, I mean, I know quite a bit about Catholicism, but maybe you can help me more. Do you believe that you will be judged for the way you've lived your life here?

Miriam: By God, you mean?

LMW: By God.

Miriam: Exactly, yes.

LMW: And so, if God were to judge you today, do you think He would be happy with you... .

Miriam: I don't know.

LMW: ...Or not happy?

Miriam: This is what I'm asking myself, you see.

LMW: AH...and what do you say to yourself?

Miriam: We all know in my family I'm afraid to die, even my children. I kept telling them, really, so many times a month, I'm afraid, I'm not afraid to be sick or something, it's to die... .

LMW: It's to die being fearful that you will be judged.

Comments about Therapeutic Conversations

After this significant disclosure and further clarification of her beliefs, I made a beginning effort to challenge this constraining belief. I attempted this by asking a question that I routinely ask in my practice: a hypothetical facilitating belief question (Wright et al., 1996). This question offers and embeds a facilitating belief and is an indirect way of challenging or altering a constraining belief. The question always begins with, "If you were to believe... ." This question invited this woman to consider an alternative facilitating belief, one suggesting that altering her beliefs may give rise to new stories and new behaviors.

LMW: This might seem like a very strange question, but I'm going to ask it anyway. If you were to believe, if you were to believe for even 10 minutes today, that God was very pleased with you, at how you've lived your life as a wife, as a mother, as a person...

Miriam: That would change everything.

LMW: ...What difference would that make in your life?

Miriam: It would change everything for me.

LMW: Can you tell me what it would change? What would be a couple of things that would change for you?

Miriam: First of all, I wouldn't be scared anymore, and then, I would say, well, if I die tomorrow; well, I die tomorrow, then I know where I would go. God knows when.

LMW: And if you weren't scared any more, how would you live your life differently, do you think? What would be different for you?

Miriam: Well, I would be more, um, calm... .

LMW: More calm...?

Miriam: Definitely, because it's all inside, it's working on me all the time and, uh, I wouldn't live that stress that I live all the time and...if you understand what I mean?

LMW: Yes, I do...if you could believe, I just want to make really sure I've got this—if you could believe even just for 10 minutes that God was pleased with you, that you had lived a good life, that He would judge you very well, you said that would make all the difference in the world for you... .

Miriam: Exactly, yes, definitely.

LMW: ...That you would be calmer, and you would be more... .

Miriam: I wouldn't be on anybody's nerves like I am on account of death.

LMW: Yes. Wow, that's incredible.

Comments about Therapeutic Conversations

Here was a woman who had suffered terribly for many years with the belief that she will have a heart attack *and* an even more troubling belief that she does not know how she will be judged when she dies. Consequently, she does not know where she will go after death.

In this next interaction, an even more amazing revelation came forth. This woman is considering discontinuing all of her antidepressant medication. Of course, this piqued my curiosity to learn that, if she were to believe she was going to heaven, would she need less medication? Her responses are astounding, and her beliefs begin to change during our evolving therapeutic conversation. Her response was even more amazing as she completed my sentence and knew exactly the connection that I was hypothesizing.

LMW: I don't know, maybe this is a crazy idea, but I'm wondering, um, do you think that if you could believe that you were going to heaven, do you think there's any connection there; that you would need... .

Miriam: ...Less pills?

LMW: Yes, that you would need less pills.

Miriam: Sure, definitely.

LMW: Wow! So maybe this idea that if you have the courage, and are more positive... .

Miriam: Yes, just like a lightning (*points to head, perhaps indicating a "light bulb"*), right?

LMW: You start to think that "Yes, I am a good person; I will probably be judged very well by God, and be able to go to heaven." And I want you to know I have similar religious beliefs about heaven... .

Miriam: You do?

LMW: ...and hell, and that we will be judged, and I hope I do okay, too, but I don't worry about it all the time like you do. That must be a terrible thing.

Miriam: Oh, it IS terrible, sometimes I used to say to Aaron, it's terrible, you don't know what I feel inside, it's like I could scream.

LMW: Yes... .

Miriam: Some days I used to say I would prefer to die, but still I said, I don't want to die.

LMW: So you think there could be a connection there. So, as you would come off the pills, maybe then you would be getting more courage about believing more positively about yourself?

Miriam: Exactly.

Comments about Therapeutic Conversations

At the end of this session, I offered my impressions and commendations to this family. I offered what I believed that I had learned from this couple, particularly from this open, courageous woman. I also related to her how I would like to tell her story to others.

LMW: I want to tell you a couple of my impressions and a couple of things that I've learned from you today! The first thing I have learned is that you've been married 38 years, and the thing that you've really taught me today is that even after 38 years of marriage, marriages can get better, it doesn't have to stay the same or get worse, right?

Miriam and Aaron: Yes, yes.

Miriam: I'm so happy about that.

LMW: That you would probably say, I'm guessing, that you would say your marriage is perhaps the best it has ever been, would you go that far?

Miriam: Exactly, yes.

LMW: One of the best... .

Miriam: For me, yes.

LMW: ...One of the best periods in your marriage... .

Aaron: Oh, yes, one of the best periods for us.

LMW: ....Periods in your marriage.

Aaron and Miriam: Definitely, yes.

LMW: See, that is incredible! After 38 years, it's even getting better! This is one thing I've really learned today, that we should never give up hope on marriages. That they can even get better, even after many, many years of marriage. The other thing that I've learned today that was very helpful to me is this notion that illness doesn't always have to be a terrible thing in a family. Illness sometimes can be scary, it can be a terrible thing, but some very good, positive things can come out of it. Your marriage is stronger, you've come together, you've united more, and that's a very wonderful thing. (*This occurred through their sessions at the outpatient nursing clinic.*) The other thing (*addressing Miriam*), is that, when I go back to Calgary, my students will be asking me, "What did you learn?" I'm going to think about you, and you know the story I would like to tell, can I tell you? ...is the story about a woman who believed for many, many years, I feel very touched by this story...but—a woman who believed for many years that she was going to maybe be judged very harshly by God. That she wasn't sure if she would go to heaven or hell, and yet, through her own courage, she made a connection that maybe she didn't need to be on antidepressant medication anymore, if she could begin to have more ideas and better beliefs about herself. That she was a very good person and a good wife and good mother. And as she started to just THINK about that a little bit, and allow herself that idea, she also came up with the idea that maybe she could give up her antidepressant medication of 20 years!!! That is a remarkable story that I would like to tell!

Comments about Therapeutic Conversation

As we said goodbye to one another, Miriam told me that she had not wanted to come to the session that day but was very grateful that she did. She also spontaneously hugged me as we bid each other goodbye. And I hugged her back.

As our conversation evolved, I believe that we experienced increasing awe, respect, and a deep emotional and spiritual connection with one another. I trust that this piece of clinical work also illustrates the phenomenon of reverencing between this courageous woman and me. I have come to believe that "reverencing" is when there is a profound awe and respect, mingled with love, for the individuals seated in front of me. This was certainly my experience with this devoted couple. (See Chapter 5 for further discussion about the phenomena of "reverencing."

Concluding Thoughts

The depth of one person's suffering is distinguished from that of others by each person's unique experience. I have ached, cried, and lamented when I have suffered with others, but it is only my own suffering that I have experienced first hand. Suffering experiences cannot be compared, but unfortunately comparisons *are* made about which sufferings we believe are the most horrific. The most important role we have as nurses is to be listeners and witnesses to others' sufferings. We must acknowledge suffering and ask questions that will challenge any constraining beliefs that may be exacerbating suffering, and we must encourage more facilitating beliefs, possibilities, and opportunities for change, growth, and healing.

Through this type of exchange between family members and nurses about suffering, a domain of spirituality is encountered. This journey into spirituality manifests itself in the offering of reverencing, compassion, and love between and among family members and nurses. Likewise, these efforts to alleviate suffering cross the border into healing, a healing that is not reserved only for family members but also includes nurses. As Frank (1995) suggests, the primary lesson that the ill have to offer us is the "pedagogy of suffering." Through this highly privileged exchange, beliefs, suffering, and spirituality become the trinity and the soul of healing in our clinical work with families. By healing, I mean "learning to live without fear, to be at peace with life, and ultimately death" (Cousins, 1989). The Trinity Model can be a useful way to conceptualize the complex concepts and interconnections of beliefs, suffering, and spirituality within the context of serious illness.

References

Cousins, N. (1989). *Beliefs become biology* (videotape). Victoria, British Columbia, Canada: University of Victoria.

Frank, A.W. (1994). Interrupted stories, interrupted lives. *Second Opinion, 20*(1), 11–18.

Frank, A.W. (1995). *The wounded storyteller: Body, illness and ethics.* Chicago: University of Chicago Press.

Hinds, C. (1992). Suffering: A relatively unexplored phenomenon among family caregivers of non-institutionalized patients with cancer. *Journal of Advanced Nursing, 17,* 918–925.

Kermode, S., & Brown, C. (1996). The postmodernist hoax and its effect on nursing. *International Journal of Nursing Studies, 33*(4), 375–384.

Sections of this chapter have been reprinted with permission from Wright, L.M. (1999). Spirituality, suffering, and beliefs: The soul of healing with families. In Walsh, F. (Ed.), *Spiritual Resources in Family Therapy.* (pp. 61–75). New York: Guilford.

Lindholm, L., & Eriksson, K. (1993). To understand and alleviate suffering in a caring culture. *Journal of Advanced Nursing, 18,* 1354–1361.

Maturana, H., & Varela, F. (1992). *The tree of knowledge: The biological roots of human understanding.* Boston, MA: Shambhala Publications, Inc.

McLain, C.S., Rosenfeld, B., & Breitbart, W. (2003). Effect of spiritual well-being on end-of-life despair in terminally-ill cancer patients. *The Lancet, 361*(9369), 1603–1607.

Morse, J.M., & Johnson, J.L. (1991). Toward a theory of illness: The Illness-Constellation Model. In J.M. Morse and J.L. Johnson (Eds.), *The illness experience: Dimensions of suffering* (pp. 315–342). Newbury Park, CA: Sage.

Moules, N.J. (2000). Postmodernism and the sacred: Reclaiming connection in our greater-than-human worlds. *Journal of Marital and Family Therapy, 2*(1), 241–253.

Patterson, R.B. (1994). Learning from suffering. *Family Therapy News,* pp. 11–12.

Tapp, D.M., & Wright, L.M. (1996). Live supervision and family systems nursing: Postmodern influences and dilemmas. *Journal of Psychiatric and Mental Health Nursing, 3*(4), 225–233.

Tomm, K. (1987). Interventive interviewing—Part II. Reflexive questioning as a means to enable self-healing. *Family Process,* 26, 167–183.

von Bertalanffy, L. (1974). General systems theory and psychiatry. In S. Arieti (Ed.), *American handbook of psychiatry* (pp. 1095–1117). New York: Basic Books.

Watson, J. (1995). Postmodernism and knowledge development in nursing. *Nursing Science Quarterly, 8,* 60–64.

Wright, L.M., & Leahey, M. (2000). *Nurses and families: A guide to family assessment and intervention* (3rd ed.). Philadelphia: F.A. Davis Co.

Wright, L.M., Watson, W.L., & Bell, J.M. (1996). *Beliefs: The heart of healing in families and illness*. New York: Basic Books.

5

Clinical Practices that Optimize Healing: Creating and Opening Space for Suffering and Spirituality in Conversations about Illness

"Florence Nightingale, who, by changing hospital conditions for victims of the Crimean War, brought about an absolute miracle. Perhaps no other woman, in the history of the world so far as I know, has done as much to reduce human misery, as this lady with the lamp, who walked through the vast wards of Scutari in the middle of the 19th century, spreading cheer and comfort, faith and hope, to those who writhed in pain. Hers was a life of excellence."

Gordon B. Hinckley

I wonder what kinds of conversations Florence Nightingale engaged in as she nursed in those wards at Scutari with suffering soldiers who were wounded and/or dying. What in particular did she say that brought comfort, hope, and possible healing? We can speculate that, with her great faith and her belief that nursing was indeed a calling from God, perhaps healing words or touch came easily to her! Or perhaps she was more mortal than we know. Maybe even Florence Nightingale had moments of wondering what to say to a 20-year-old dying soldier who was worrying about the great suffering his death would bring to his mother, or another young man in great pain and suffering because of his shot-off limbs. Nightingale writes, "...the first idea I can recollect when I was a child was a desire to nurse the sick. My day dreams were all of hospitals and I visited them whenever I could" (Dossey, 2000).

The simple desire to nurse and to care for others in times of suffering from illness is an honorable and sufficient foundation from which to build more deliberate and conscious therapeutic conversations that are conducive to telling illness narratives that open space for suffering and spirituality.

This chapter offers some clinical guideposts and a road map for the kinds of conversations about suffering and spirituality that nurses can encourage to offer possibilities for healing. How these ideas can be applied in clinical practice by using the Trinity Model (see Chapter 4) are presented, and specific clinical guideposts are offered in a clinical example drawn from my practice and research at the Family Nursing Unit (FNU) at the University of Calgary. Families have acknowledged that these clinical guideposts have been useful in reducing their suffering.

Clinical Guideposts

In my clinical work with individuals and families experiencing serious illness, I believe that my goal and obligation are to alleviate or diminish emotional, physical, or spiritual suffering. Some of the guideposts or interventions that I have found useful to alleviate or diminish suffering are acknowledging suffering and the sufferer; inviting, listening to, and witnessing stories of suffering; recognizing and challenging my constraining beliefs; creating a healing context for reducing suffering; inviting reflections about suffering; reverencing and loving; and prayer and praying. These guideposts are by no means all inclusive, but are simply one road map for the care of persons with serious illness.

GUIDEPOST 1: ACKNOWLEDGING SUFFERING AND THE SUFFERER

One beginning effort to alleviate suffering is to acknowledge that it exists. Suffering is frequently the total sum of the illness experience, whether

it is short and intense or prolonged and perva-
sive. Suffering is part of our human existence,
from stories like that of Job in the Judeo-
Christian faith; to stories of Holocaust victims;
to stories of illness, disability, and loss. These
stories belong to sufferers! The acknowledgment of the sufferer and the experience of
suffering by health-care providers can be a powerful starting point to begin understanding and
healing. Comments such as "This time in your
life is really tough" or "What your family is experiencing is a real tragedy" or "I can only imagine
how difficult this must be for all of you" are examples of acknowledging sufferers and their suffering. After acknowledging and validating one
couple's experience with the serious illness of
their infant, the mother responded to me, "This
is the first time that any health professional has
seemed to appreciate what a difficult and stressful time we have had. They talk to us as if life is
normal, except you have an ill child. But life is
not normal and has not been normal for a long,
long time." A man, when I acknowledged his suffering from leukemia, said to me, "It is good to
hear that you say we have been through a tough
time because it has been very tough, but it really
helps to know that someone else realizes that."
These are only a couple of examples of the numerous times that patients and families have responded in kind when it was acknowledged that
they were living in the midst of suffering. The deliberate and clear acknowledgment of suffering
frequently opens the door for the disclosure of

other fears or worries not previously expressed, such as the fear of a caregiver who was worried about who would care for her spouse if her health failed. Nurses can use this guidepost in positive and productive ways.

GUIDEPOST 2: INVITING, LISTENING TO, AND WITNESSING STORIES OF SUFFERING

Inviting, listening to, and witnessing stories of illness and suffering provide a powerful validation of an important human experience. Health professionals are in a privileged position to hear and affirm illness narratives. By inviting the telling of illness stories, we engage in the essential, ethical practice of recognizing the ill person as the "suffering other" (Frank, 1994). In my clinical practice, I also want to open possibilities, through therapeutic conversations, for recognizing the ill person and other family members as the heroic other, the joyful other, the giving other, the receiving other, the compassionate other, the passionate other, and the strengthened other (Wright, Watson, & Bell, 1996).

Positive responses from family members to our interventions and a reduction in emotional, physical, and spiritual suffering have convinced me of the necessity to invite family members to tell their illness stories. In our professional encounters with families, we move beyond social conversations about the illness to purposeful therapeutic conversations. We direct the conversation in a manner that we hope will give voice to the human experiences of suffering and symptoms as well as to the experiences of courage, hope, growth, and love. Through the telling of the story, "the patient can interpret her own suffering (and, I would add, strength); the role of witness is to provide moral affirmation of the struggle to find that interpretation. Thus the patient's voice must be cultivated, not cut off" (Frank, 1994, p. 14).

By providing a context for the sharing among family members of their illness experiences, intense emotions are legitimized. By inviting family members to share their illness narratives, which include stories of sickness and suffering, we allow them, as Frank (1994) suggests, to reclaim their right to tell their own experiences and to reclaim a voice over the medical voice and a life beyond illness. Kleinman (1988) proffered the idea that an inquiry into the meanings (beliefs) of illness is a journey into relationships. I have had many families tell me that having someone listen to their stories, ask questions about their stories, and commend them for their courage in the face of suffering has enabled them to gain a new and sometimes renewed appreciation of their ability to cope. Through this witnessing, listening, and commending, the family's resilience is often rediscovered with very positive outcomes. In many instances, these positive outcomes have been the alleviation of physical symptoms and familial conflict as well as emotional and/or spiritual suffering.

One of our most difficult duties as human beings is to listen to the voices of those who suffer. The voices of the ill are easy to ignore, because these voices are often faltering in tone and mixed in message... . Listening is hard, but it is also a fundamental moral act; to realize the best potential in postmodern times requires an ethics of listening. The moment of witness in the story crystallizes a mutuality of need, when each is *for* the other. (Frank, 1995, p. 25)

One of the more famous stories of suffering is the biblical story of Job. In this story, Job suffers many afflictions that neither he nor his friends can understand. On seeing Job, his friends can barely speak to or recognize him.

And when they lifted up their eyes afar off, and knew him not, they lifted up their voice and wept; and they rent every one his mantle, and sprinkled dust upon their heads toward heaven.

So they sat down with him upon the ground seven days and seven nights, and none spake a word unto him: for they saw that his suffering was very great.

Job 2: 12–13, *Holy Bible, King James Version*

At first, his friends were indeed compassionate, in the sense of compassion meaning "to suffer with." But unfortunately, they were not compassionate for long. After the 7 days and nights, Eliphaz the Temanite began blaming Job for his own troubles. Attempting to guess the reasons for Job's troubles, they were a bit more like enemies than friends.

Inherent in the experience of suffering is often the sense of being isolated or alone, a sense of being different or set apart. Being "set apart" in suffering seems to invite such conclusions, not only from friends and family but also from the sufferers themselves. Our inclination is to recoil in the face of suffering, our own or others. Job's friends recoiled as they turned to blame him for his troubles. In this maneuver, they distanced themselves and attempted to assert some measure of control over suffering. If Job can be seen to have caused his own suffering, they are safe. They can control their own possible loss of health and possible immersion in suffering (McLeod, 2003, p. 160).

By inviting, listening to, and witnessing stories of suffering, we are not recoiling, retreating, or reneging on our obligation to listen to the voices of those who suffer. So how do we invite these stories of illness? We do so through the asking of questions such as, "Tell me how this illness has changed your life," "I'm curious as to what you believe has been the reaction of your family members to your illness," "What has been the greatest surprise with your illness?," "What has been the effect on your marriage, your children, of this illness," or "What are you most concerned about with your illness?" These questions are invitations to hear and listen to how illness has affected individual and family lives. It provides an opportunity for health professionals to give the gift of deep listening and to create a reverencing connection through the moral obligation to respond to suffering.

I have discovered in my clinical practice that, when a person is suffering, his or her internal conversations are usually filled with questions. To externalize these internalized conversations, I ask questions such as "What questions do you find yourself asking these days?" "What questions do you ask on a good day/on a bad day?" "Have you received an answer to these questions?" "Do you need an answer?" "What if you never receive an answer?" "Do you pray; if so, what do you pray for?" These kinds of questions are entry points into the world of sufferers. Frequently, these internalized questions have not been spoken before, and by externalizing them, clients report that it begins to reduce the intensity of their suffering.

GUIDEPOST 3: RECOGNIZING AND CHALLENGING OUR OWN CONSTRAINING BELIEFS ABOUT SUFFERING

Health professionals' beliefs can hinder or enhance the possibilities for alleviating suffering (Levac, McLean, Wright, and Bell, 1998; Wright, Bell, Watson, & Tapp, 1995). One belief frequently offered to those suffering with illness is that "life could be worse." This belief is benevolently offered to provide comfort and encouragement. One woman, suffering from endometriosis, did not find this belief useful. She responded: "I know life could be worse. I could have only one eye or leg, and I am very fortunate to have all I do have.... . But those philosophies do not solve the disease, do not get rid of the pain, the tears, the frustrations, or the heartaches that come with the problems" (Donoghue & Siegel, 1992, p. 55). This example highlights the need for health professionals to recognize that each person's suffering with illness is unique and that attempting to have persons "count their blessings" can inadvertently trivialize suffering from illness. Often persons who are spared from dying after a life-threatening illness or accident still find that their lives and relationships are dramatically altered and changed and are given direct and indirect messages by well-meaning health professionals that they should be thankful and grateful that things were not worse—"at least you are here." We, as health professionals, need to challenge such beliefs and recognize that we cannot judge what should make life meaningful and purposeful for another. Rather, we need to assist others to embrace life and find meaning and purpose that is meaningful to them.

GUIDEPOST 4: CREATING A HEALING CONTEXT FOR REDUCING SUFFERING

The ultimate desired outcome is to create a healing context or environment for family members for the relief of suffering from their illness experiences. By *healing*, we mean "learning to live without fear, to be at peace with life, and ultimately death" (Cousins, 1989). Remen (1993) eloquently offered the following notion:

Healing is different from curing. Healing is a
process we're all involved in all the time... .
Sometimes people heal physically, and they don't
heal emotionally, or mentally, or spiritually. And
sometimes people heal emotionally, and they
don't heal physically. (p. 244)

Frank (1995) offers the powerful metaphor
that ill people are more than victims of disease
or patients of medicine—they are wounded storytellers. He argues that people tell stories to
make sense of their suffering; when they turn
their diseases into stories, they find healing.

This coincides with a strong belief that exists
in our North American health-care culture that
eliciting, discussing, and expressing one's illness
story and accompanying emotions can be very
healing (Wright et al, 1996). Families have often
remarked in my clinical practice how they appreciated the opportunity to talk about their illness
experiences and the healing effect these conversations had on their lives and relationships.

One young man in his 30s was suffering with
chronic pain from multiple sclerosis. When I explored the deterioration in his condition since
our last meeting, he told me he was experiencing much more severe pain in his chest and
hands. But as I invited him to reflect on his increased suffering, he told me about his beliefs
regarding treatment for the pain, which were fascinating. He did not believe that traditional medication was helping or alleviating his chronic
pain. In fact, he reported that it made him "feel
strange." Nor was he prepared to take any more
steroid treatments. Rather, he told me that he

had found some relief from his pain "by smoking an occasional joint." When I inquired about his beliefs regarding what he thought might be triggering these recent multiple sclerosis attacks and the subsequent increased suffering with pain, he said that he believed it was the stress of his current divorce proceedings and having to move from his present home. He later told me that my question invited him for the first time to make this connection between his suffering from chronic pain and his divorce, and this connection seemed to have a positive influence on reducing his chronic pain.

The capacity of health professionals to be "witnesses" to the stories of suffering of patients and families is central to providing care; it is frequently the genesis of healing, if not curing (Frank, 1994; Kleinman, 1988).

GUIDEPOST 5: INVITING REFLECTIONS ABOUT SUFFERING

To alter existing beliefs, health professionals need to invite family members to a reflection about their constraining beliefs (Wright et al., 1996). Through these reflections, a person begins to entertain different or alternative beliefs to get out of a state of confusion, struggle, or suffering. For example, beliefs about hope and optimism in the illness experience have generally not been addressed by the dominant medical system. Consequently, the appeal of complementary, integrative, or alternative healing approaches becomes very understandable. Many

persons suffering with illness find these approaches more positive than the conventional
medical approach because the complementary
healing approaches do not shy away from some
of the big questions surrounding illness: Why has
this illness happened to me? Why do people get
sick despite living well? Why do some people die
"before their time?" Why is my condition becoming worse?

Another woman who was seen in the FNU was
facing a double tragedy. Both her husband and
her 10-year-old son had life-threatening illnesses.
When asked about the impact of this on her life,
she responded, "I myself am not afraid to die; I
am afraid of living. How can I go on without the
two people whom I love the most?" The ultimate
goal, of course, is that, through reflection, individuals and family members will find other ways
to understand their suffering, make meaning of
their suffering, and ultimately regain hope and
resilience for their futures. This courageous
woman found meaning in her faith, although it
was fragile for a time, to find meaning in her suffering.

We can also learn and invite reflections about
various clients' and family members' spiritual
and religious beliefs that may or may not contribute to their suffering. For example, a health
professional might inquire, "What are the beliefs
of your Muslim (or Sufi, Buddhist, North
American native, Jewish, Christian, or other)
faith that help or hinder your suffering right
now? What do Muslims believe is the reason for
suffering? Do you agree with that belief? Has

your experience with your illness strengthened or challenged that belief?"

GUIDEPOST 6: REVERENCING AND LOVING

In recent years, I have had one recurring piece of feedback about my clinical work with families that has guided me in becoming more cognizant and appreciative of the spiritual dimension of therapeutic conversations. Colleagues and students alike have been offering their unsolicited observations on the "spiritual" aspects of my clinical work for many years. I found this observation fascinating because I had not put any direct or intended emphasis on spiritual issues in my clinical work. I reflected that somehow I must have changed from my early years as a clinician because this feedback was news of a difference (Bateson, 1979). The greatest reflection came after a valued colleague told me that he would describe my clinical work as "secular theology." This comment perturbed me for some time. He elaborated and suggested what he believed to be the most powerful aspect of my clinical work. This colleague offered the thought that what occurred between clients, family members, and myself was the phenomenon of *reverencing*. When we open space to the comments of others about ourselves personally and professionally, they are often followed by great reflections. I pondered this observation for some time and reflected on the meaning of reverence. I have come to believe that "reverencing" occurs when there is a profound awe and respect, mingled with love, for the individuals seated in front of me. I often feel that same reverencing from clients and family members being returned to me.

In these moments of reverencing in clinical work, something very special happens between the nurse and the individual or family; it is something felt by all—a deep emotional connection. I know and have felt these moments in clinical work, whether directly in the room with the family or from behind a one-way mirror as a supervisor or team member. During these times, I have witnessed the most profound changes in family members' thinking, behavior, illness experience, and, most important, their suffering. In these instances, I have felt an emotion that seems to arise only when there is reverencing. This emotion, I submit, is pure love. I have come to understand and recognize moments of reverencing as one dimension or aspect of the spiritual nature of my clinical work with families that perhaps invites colleagues and students to comment that they observe "spiritual" aspect to my work with families. I hope this is so, because I believe it makes a quantum difference to the healing process when reverencing occurs.

Since I have received this very significant feedback and reflection on my clinical work, it has now been my routine practice for the past few years to explore "spiritual" issues and practices and to be more aware of this particular way of dealing with clients and families who are experiencing serious illness.

GUIDEPOST 7: PRAYER
AND PRAYING

The quiet intervention of prayer is also receiving more attention in my clinical work with families. Dossey (1993) reviewed numerous medical studies examining the efficacy of prayer in producing physical changes. For example, he suggested that the ritual of prayer may trigger emotions that, in turn, may lead to changes in health by having a positive effect on the immune and cardiovascular systems. Thomas (1997) conducted a fascinating review of physicians who pray for or with their patients and who encourage their patients to pray for themselves and within their religious community. From this review, he offered his belief that some prayer is better than no prayer.

McNeil (1998) found that, when hospitalized patients experiencing pain were given a pain questionnaire to complete, 76 percent cited personal prayer as being the most commonly used nondrug method for pain management. Dossey (1993) and Cousins (1989) summoned health professionals to recognize that there are many nonphysiological reasons that persons and families heal from illness. Prayer in my daily personal life is a well-established ritual. Over the past few years, I have on occasion adopted Dossey's (1993) practice of praying for, although not with, the clients and families with whom I work.

As Dossey (1993) suggested, if a health professional believes that prayer works, not to use it is analogous to withholding a potent medication or surgical procedure:

 Both prayer and belief are nonlocal manifestation of consciousness, because both can operate at a distance, sometimes outside the patient's awareness. Both affirm that "it's not all physical," and both can be used as an adjunct to other forms of therapy. (p. 141)

In praying for our clients, we perhaps also heighten our connection with them and our investment in their recovery and well-being. I also find it useful to ask individuals and families, "Do you pray? If so, what do you pray for?"

CLINICAL PRACTICE EXAMPLE: "WILL I EVER BE WHOLE AGAIN?"

I offer a therapeutic narrative that transpired between a loving and courageous husband and wife, Bill and Myrna (51 and 47 years old, respectively), and our clinical team at the FNU. This therapeutic narrative highlights how conversations about suffering and spirituality can be brought forth, explored, invited, and distinguished to, we hope, invoke healing. This couple was referred to our outpatient clinic by their family physician. One of our Masters of Nursing students, Juliet Thornton, was the clinician with this family. Other members of the clinical team consisted of graduate nursing students and two faculty supervisors, of whom one was myself. In total, we had five sessions with this couple and their two adult sons, who attended two of the

sessions. At the time of referral, Bill was experiencing the aftermath of a stroke and was in
remission with leukemia. Unfortunately, Bill's
stroke occurred during his chemotherapy
treatment for the leukemia. He was noticeably
affected by this stroke with a number of neuro-
logical deficits, including some difficulty with
speech, cognition, and left-sided weakness in
both his arm and leg. Bill was no longer able to
teach in the public school system, which he
had enjoyed so much for 27 years.

In the first meeting with individuals or families,
we make it a routine practice to ask them a
question that I have called the "one-question
question" (Wright, 1989). Specifically, "If there
was just one question that you could have answered during our work together, what would
that one question be?" By asking this question,
I believe that we are often able to identify the
area of greatest suffering. Frequently, this is NOT
the particular presenting concern. The responses
to this question, I believe, come from a different
place, and a deeper place within a person than
is answered by simply asking the question,
"What is your greatest concern?" Of course, this
question is also useful for identifying potential
emotional or spiritual suffering, and is more appropriate in the beginning stages of a meeting.
We have learned in our practice that it seems
more fitting to ask the "one-question question"
toward the end of a first meeting with an individual or family members once a beginning therapeutic relationship has begun.

It became apparent that Bill had many questions about his future that were causing great suffering as a result of such losses at the young age of 51 compounded by no apparent answers that brought relief or meaning. One of the concerns that was uppermost in his mind was whether his physical progress had gone as far as it could, and therefore should he accept it, or would there be further recovery? Health-care providers understandably were reluctant to give any definitive answers to this aspect of his recovery. But this situation of "not knowing" had sunk Bill into a place of hopelessness, depression, and weeping. Myrna fell into the interactional trap that many spouses, as well as health-care providers, fall into: what I refer to as the "cheer-up phenomenon." The more a loved one or client shows sadness or discouragement, the more cheering up and encouraging is done. Frequently, these well-intended acts of kindness to "cheer up" another only enhance the suffering rather than diminish it because the person's suffering is not validated, but rather walked over, ignored, or minimized. Myrna also wondered what the future held for her husband and queried her role in this dilemma of "pushing or not pushing," encouraging or not encouraging her husband to do more. In the therapeutic dialogue that follows, notice how quickly we learn the impact and influence of this illness on all family members. Illness and the suffering that are embedded within it are indeed a family affair. (JT indicates Juliet Thornton, the Masters student who was the nurse interviewer with this family.)

First Session

Myrna: Like do we just wait? Do we wait for Bill to get out of that space or should I be pushing him? Should he be trying more—is it normal to do what he's doing or should we be pushing him more? Or should we not push him and just leave him the way that he is? This is really affecting our family. It's hard for both of us and for our sons. You never realize the difference.

Bill: It is catastrophic… .

Myrna: Yeah. Like people think that he's so lucky that he's come through and he's done so well. And he has. But it changes your whole life.

Bill: Yeah… .

Myrna: Like I'll say to him, "it could be worse, you know," but that doesn't seem to help. Because, you know, it could be a lot worse. Maybe he wouldn't be walking or talking or anything else. But that doesn't help him. He just has a lot of trouble dealing with what he has left.

Bill: I don't know whether you can provide me with strategies, um, how do you get a person to accept the way they are? I don't know whether that's just something I'm going to have to work on. Maybe I'm going too fast. Maybe I expect too much. I don't know.

JT: So what I'm hearing now, and this can change as we work together, is that you would like some advice on how to live in this space that you're experiencing right now?

Myrna: Yeah. Are we doing the right thing or the wrong thing?

JT: OK.

Myrna: Is it—like I don't know. Sometimes I think I want to push him and I want to shake him and say,

"At least you're here." And other times I understand it's so hard for him. It's fine to say, "Well, at least you can still walk," but the fact that he can't use his arm and his speech is impaired—I guess in terms of, am I doing the right thing? Should I just leave him alone? But when I try to do that I feel that's wrong. I should be encouraging him.

JT: And so your hope really is to find some strategies to learn to live with Bill's condition?

Bill: Yeah. Like I don't know what the future is going to hold and that really bothers me because—what is going to happen? Like am I just going to continue this way throughout my life, like just veg? Or what am I going to do? I just—I don't know.

Myrna: Like when he gets really—like he will sit and cry—"What's to become of me?" And that breaks my heart when I hear him like that. I felt that way when he was sick and I thought is this going to be our life, you know? It's scary. Nobody thought he would come this far but will it ever come all the way back? When do you give up and accept that "this is as good as it gets"? You never give up. But nobody gives any answers.

JT: And what do you (looking at Bill) think about Myrna's thoughts about what the future holds?

Bill: Yeah, I agree with her. I don't know whether I should get pushed more. Half of me says I should be thankful and just take each day as it comes, but when you're used to having a life and I don't have much of a life. It just seems more and more (weeping) has been taken away from me—my teaching, my driver's license—it just keeps adding up. So I don't know whether to try or I don't know whether to give up. Am I beating myself against a wall (weeping)? Should I accept the way it is? But I don't want to accept that.

Comments/Reflections

Indeed, life has lost all meaning for Bill. It is now a life of contradictions, dilemmas, and great suffering. The poignancy of his suffering is almost palpable, even in the pages of this text. His suffering is magnified as his beliefs are challenged and altered, as exemplified by his comment: "half of me says that I should be thankful...but I don't have much of a life." The numerous losses Bill has experienced impede his ability to be grateful for his life because they invite him to think what has been lost, and therefore, what IS the purpose of his life now? This lack of purpose and meaning for his life connects his suffering to issues of spirituality. The conceptualization of the Trinity Model is readily apparent and useful here because Bill's beliefs, suffering, and spirituality are so closely intertwined. This is now where beliefs, suffering, and spirituality begin to connect.

Second Session

In the second session, the suffering centered around Bill's condition emerged again. But it is incredibly difficult to listen to stories of suffering. However, I harbor a profound belief that talking is healing, particularly talking about suffering from illness. I also believe that this healing occurs not just in the emotional domain but also in the physical domain. Many, many individuals and families over the years have shared with our clinical team how their physical symptoms have diminished or disappeared when they experienced reduced suffering. Our clinical team has also observed these phenomena because they are so evident in the change in the faces of sufferers. Reduced suffering results in distinct physiological changes.

I also believed that Bill needed to be able to tell his illness narrative fully without being interrupted, cheered up, or stopped in his storytelling. Knowing that this would be a difficult task for our young clinician, Juliet, I made a supervisory phone-in (intercom phone-in system between myself as supervisor and the clinician) to offer some direction and support to the student. I pointed out the interactional pattern between Bill's suffering and Myrna's attempts to cheer him up. Every time Bill expressed any verbal or nonverbal suffering, Myrna would interrupt by attempting to cheer him up and Bill would then become silent and suffer more internally, which in turn invited Myrna to continue her efforts to cheer him up, and thus the cycle continued. I asked this young, compassionate clinician to just listen to Bill's story, without interruption, without further questions, without any immediate reflection. Juliet beautifully implemented this phone-in and even took it a step further by requesting, most gently, of Myrna, that BOTH she and Juliet would "just listen" to Bill. This was a very different experience for both Myrna and Bill. Bill's speaking was preceded by almost a minute of silence and deep, deep sighing on his part. This was a prelude to allowing his suffering to come forward, and come forward it did.

JT: I guess I would just like to invite both of us, myself and you, Myrna, to kind of sit back and let you (Bill) talk about your situation and what you're thinking. So if that's okay, we'll just be quiet and listen and then you can tell us when we can talk.

Mryna: You just say what you feel.
(Bill sighed several times and there was a long period of silence. Neither the clinician Juliet nor Myrna spoke. Then Bill began his tale of suffering.)

Bill: Some days I just feel—well, it is really hard—it is hard accepting the way things are. I tell myself that I should—that I should be thankful that I'm alive—that these things have happened to me and I have to accept them, but I just get really frustrated that I cannot do things like I used to. I trip over things. I understand that my brain doesn't work the way it used to (silence). I sit on my balcony and I see people walking and riding and walking their dogs without looking like a gimp, and I am a gimp (sobbing). I don't know what I'm going to do. I think a lot about that. I can't take each day as it comes and live life being thankful that I didn't die. I have Myrna here with me. But so much is unknown. I know it sounds silly 'cause there is always the unknown but at least like Myrna knows she's going to work; she's got her job—she's got this, she's got that. I *don't* know. And, you know, you come here (referring to Juliet) and talk to us and things like that. You've got some sort of schedule to your life. Like my doctor said she'd die to have 2 weeks off. I, uh, I do not know what my future is going to hold and I think a lot about that. Maybe I should not; I don't know. (Pause) If I could do something beneficial. I just do not want to spend my time getting up, making the bed, doing the dishes, doing the laundry. Like I don't mind doing that—it is not like I hate it. But there has got to be something more. And it is just coming to accept that. I guess it is going to take—well, I know it is going to take time. But—I just, uh—(sighing). Am I making any sense?

JT: Yes. Is it okay, Bill, if we talk?

Bill: Sure.

JT: Okay. I am just wondering what you (Myrna) are thinking as you listen?

Myrna: I just feel his pain and I know that he—if you could have known what he was like before his illness and how just the kind of person that he is, you would realize how difficult this is for him. And I just can feel his pain. And I feel so helpless because—but when he is like this at home, we can talk about it, but sometimes he won't talk. It is just the same thing but I do not understand, I do not know what to do. When he gets like this—I know what he is going through in a sense because I feel it—we are a part of each other and just like he feels my pain, I feel his. And I hate leaving him some days. And I come home at lunchtime and he cries and it takes everything I have to go back to work. It takes everything I have. And these little jaunts where I take a couple of days off—like I went back to work January 24th and I have not taken a sick day since I returned to work 'cause I was off from June until January. When I get overtired or for vacation or whatever I used to have these extra days off with him so that we can do things. Even things as mundane as doing chores, but it is together.

JT: Well.

Comments/Reflections

At this point, I again called Juliet on the intercom system and offered a couple of suggestions for questions that could be asked. Juliet then shared my questions with the couple.

JT: The team just had a couple of questions. They are just wondering if you believe that talking is healing for you?

Bill: Yes and no. I look forward to these sessions. It's good to talk. It's good to get the feelings out. 'Cause if I am just with Myrna I know that I don't always talk. But, um, I do not (crying), I don't see any future for me.

Myrna: You described it as a vicious circle.

Bill: Yes, it is a vicious circle and I go around and around and around 'cause I do not see any end near. 'Cause sometimes I think this is what my whole life is going to be. Right now I do not see answers. People haven't got answers for me. Like I don't know, maybe I am rushing too much. I am off (work) until the beginning of January and then I'll see the doctor. Um— I'm anxious to get going on doing something. I have got to feel that there is some meaning to my life. I don't know. The other day I was thinking about the kids—about teaching—'bout my classroom. That is not there for me anymore. 'Cause I know I won't be able to go back teaching but (sighing) there's got to be something more. I don't know. It's a vicious circle.

Comments/Reflections

Talking is healing. But it is not rambling, undirected talking. It is talking that has occurred when a healing context has been created, when reverencing has occurred among Juliet, Bill, and Myrna and when the illness story has been invited in a particular kind of way that enables healing to begin. The telling of this illness narrative with all its embedded suffering was the *first* time that Bill had been invited to relate his story of suffering and strength. This was a pivotal and profound moment in the therapeutic sessions. A space was created for Bill's suffering to come forth by the manner in which Juliet and Myrna listened to his story without judgment, without a need to respond, without further questions, and without attempts to cheer him up. It is this kind of listening and witnessing that creates the possibility for healing to occur. But what a gift for all!

At the end of each session at the FNU, the family is offered the opportunity to listen to the ideas and reflections of our clinical nursing team. If they desire to hear the team, then we ask if there are any questions they have for the team or that they would like the team to address. We refer to this process as the Reflecting Team (Anderson, 1987). Then the clinical team comes into the interviewing room, and the family goes behind the one-way mirror to listen and observe, and have their own reflections while the team is discussing their situation. The one question that Bill wanted the team to consider was, "Will I ever be whole again?" whereas Myrna's question was "Are we heading down the right path? Is there anything else out there that can help?" Following is part of the verbatim discussion during the Reflecting Team. The clinical team consisted of graduate nursing students,

Dr. Janice M. Bell (JMB), and myself (LMW) as faculty supervisors.

Reflecting Team Discussion

LMW: So do we feel brave enough to tackle this very difficult question they are asking? So Bill was asking "Will I be whole again?" and earlier he was asking "Should I be accepting"—was that the question? "Should I be accepting this or should I be pushing myself more?" That seems like a dilemma throughout the whole interview, wasn't it? And then for Myrna it was "Are we heading down the right path?" Did she have a question earlier?

JT: Well, advice—she was wondering about advice for how to live in this space, she called it.

LMW: I mean, one of the things they are saying is that nobody can tell them? They're saying they want to know is this as far as I can go. Or can I go further?

JMB: Or should I push myself?

LMW: Or should I push myself further? And I guess I would like to not give them the party line again today and say we don't know how you're going to progress. I am willing to step out on a limb. And I would like to say that I think he *can* go farther. That I think he *should* push himself. Because I think not pushing himself is not healthy for him right now. He does not feel good about that. I think he should push himself and test his limits to see what he is capable of. Instead of waiting for the health professionals to say, "Yes, you are going to get better" or "you are not." No. Let him discover.

JMB: Well, it sounds like they have had lots of really interesting experiences already of challenging health-care professional beliefs about even whether Bill was going to live.

LMW: Yes. Health professionals try to be responsible and prepare you on one hand (for a shortened life) but miracles happen—if they think of this as a miracle. So I am saying now he has survived, for what purpose and for how far he can go I do not know that. But I do know—I do believe very strongly that he should push himself. That he should push beyond and not wait for an answer from someone else. That he should decide his own limits. And another thing that I want to offer them I learned from a woman who was a quadriplegic who was in a terrible car accident. She was a psychologist and taught a workshop that I went to. And she taught me something that's been very useful to me in my work with families. She said that you never—when health professionals are suggesting you should accept this—she said you never have to accept it. You never have to accept what has happened to you. But you do have to adjust to it. And I think that is a wonderful distinction. Bill may never want to accept that he does not have the full use of his right hand. That he maybe has some memory problems from time to time. That his right leg does not work as it once did. He never has to fully accept that. But he *does* have to adjust to it. That is what I'm saying. But adjust to what? He does not know the limits yet because he is waiting for somebody to give him direction about how far to go. And I am saying push the limits. Go for it. See how far you can go.

JMB: I take it that you think the uncertainty about that invites inertia in him?

LMW: Yes, it invites inertia, and I think it invites his depression. I think it invites him to feel very emotional, wondering, "Is this as good as it gets or is it not?" Should he accept it or should he not? I am saying he does not have to accept it. It is a terrible thing that has happened to him. It is a tragedy. He is right, at 51 years old. And so my answer, I guess, to Myrna's question is the same. When she is asking, "Should I be encouraging, should I be pushing him?" I say, push him. Get in there and let us see what he is capable of. And no more of this sitting around and trying to figure out "Should we just sit here and accept it or should we not?" I mean I just think this man has got a lot to offer. I do not know where he will end up finding himself. Maybe he will end up being at home on his computer doing interesting things—writing. Maybe he will want to get a part-time job. Maybe he will want to get full-time work somewhere. I do not know but I think he will not know that until he pushes more. But I am curious about the rest of you (asking other team members). What do you think? Do you perhaps disagree with what I am saying? Is there another way to look at that?

Nursing Student: I get the impression that he is already starting to push himself. Just doing all the work at home. I mean all the courage it takes for a man to accept or adjust to that. To do it and to learn to do the cooking like Myrna was mentioning. I think it is another way to push himself. Because it was probably not something that he was very pleased about at the beginning but now he is doing it. And also, like Myrna was mentioning, now he is going to the computer, even though she is worried that he is spending all his time on the computer looking for answers. I think it is another way to push.

LMW: Yes, that is true.

Nursing Student: She even mentioned that the time

that he is at the computer, his attention is there. He feels better looking for more answers, but at some point maybe he will say, "Okay, I can see then that I cannot get an answer," or he is going to get an answer that is going to fit for him and he will push himself a bit more. But for me, what I saw today, I really had the impression that both of them are already pushing.

LMW: You are right. Maybe he has already started.

JT: Well, I think he is very determined and creative.

Comments/Reflections

I took a very strong position in offering my own beliefs about what might be helpful for Bill. Was it a useful position to take? The proof is in the pudding. Immediately after the team's discussion, the family is invited back into the interviewing room and the team returns to its position behind the one-way mirror. Now the viewing angles are shifted once again, as the team now listens to the family's reflections on the team's reflections. We encourage the clinician to now ask the family, "What stood out for you?" as a means of knowing of all the ideas that were offered, which of the ideas "fit" with the person's biopsychosocial-spiritual structure (Maturana & Varela, 1992). In other words, which comments, opinions, or offerings by the team invited a reflection in that particular person. Change that occurs through reflection, as we have learned in our clinical practice, provides the most sustaining and powerful change. "The moment of reflection...is the moment when we become aware of that part of ourselves which we cannot see in any other way" (Maturana & Varela, 1992, p. 23). A reflection can be about the past, present, or future. It does not just mean looking back. Reflections on the present and future can be powerful influences as well.

Bill's response to my suggestion to "push the limits" was one of the comments he reported to Juliet (following the team's discussion) that he found most useful. For Bill, this was his most significant reflection. The importance of having time to think was emphasized by Andersen (1991), who was the innovator of the formal concept of the reflecting team. Other questions could also have invited a reflection, such as "If you never push yourself, what do you predict your life will be like in 6 months?" or "Do you think being in a dilemma about pushing yourself adds or diminishes stress on your body?" In addition to questions, we can invite others to a reflection by offering ideas, advice, and suggestions that can serve as useful perturbations (Wright & Levac, 1992). Of course, most nurses work independently and do not have the benefit of a reflecting team, but learning how to ask reflexive questions and offering our best professional knowledge through advice and opinions can be equally as useful. It is only when nurses are invested in the outcome (that is, expecting someone to follow our advice or believing our opinion is the correct one) that there is a likelihood that minimal or no change will occur. Anderson (1991) noted that when someone believes he can instruct another, the other defends himself and is actually less open. Maturana offers a similar belief: "You will never be able to do instructive interaction. The most that you can do is to talk to the patient and invite this person to a reflection that will allow the realization that there is an illness... . Understanding cannot be forced" (Maturana, 1998). With invitations to reflection, the challenging of constraining beliefs that invite suffering commences. Bill was suffering dreadfully with his constraining belief that perhaps he should just accept what has happened to him. By inviting Bill and Myrna to a reflection, the "truth" of their stance, which was a constrained solution (not pushing himself), is now challenged. It was now possible to offer, entice, and invite them to a differing belief that may have the possibility of reducing suffering and giving his life more meaning (Wright et al,1996). We cannot make people believe something different. We cannot *give* them a new facilitating belief. It happens through the process of mutual reverencing between the nurse and client and invitations to reflection.

This family has graciously given me permission to use the therapeutic narratives in written publications, professional conferences, and research. However, I have changed their names for reasons of confidentiality. They also participated in Dr. Deborah McLeod's (2003) hermeneutic inquiry research study to explore the meaning of spirituality and spiritual care practices in family systems nursing. In a research interview with McLeod some 2 years after our clinical work was completed, they again reported that the most

useful aspect of their five sessions at the FNU
was the advice to "push the limits" (McLeod,
2003). Myrna also commented on her experience with the team at the FNU in being invited to
"push the limits." Myrna found herself seeking
spiritual answers. She attributed this seeking to
the listening and questioning of the team. Part of
this very revealing, informative, and helpful research interview after the completion of our clinical work with this couple, which occurred with
Dr. McLeod (DM), is offered below (McLeod,
2003, p. 168).

DM: So it was the idea of pushing the limits that you
both found the most helpful?

Myrna: Yes, pushing the limits was the biggest thing,
but also looking inside yourself for the answers.

DM: Can you tell me a little bit about that?

Myrna: Well, instead of looking to the outside for answers, they encouraged us to look to the inside.

DM: Can you say something about how they did that?

Myrna: Well, when we discussed our spiritual beliefs,
they supported those and they followed through and
asked more questions, which made you think more
about your own beliefs. Their beliefs didn't come
into it. They didn't try to direct you towards their beliefs or any other beliefs. They listened to what you
believed. They accepted that and supported it and
questioned it to bring it out more which makes you
think about it more.

Bill: We definitely did more thinking about it.

Myrna: Yeah. The fact that they brought our beliefs
into the discussion and that they found our beliefs
interesting and that they were accepting of it, you

know. That made me more comfortable to be able to talk about it. I was surprised at how they wanted to discuss that aspect of our lives.

Comments/Reflections

Anderson (1991a) made a distinction between "inner talk" and "outer talk." He stated that "When we take part in the 'talking cure' we should ask ourselves all the time: is the talk I have with this person slow enough so that the other person and I have time enough for our 'inner talks?'" (p. 29). Invitations to reflection should allow time for "inner talks" and time to reflect on them.

Previously, Bill and Myrna had refused visits from clergy, believing (rightly or wrongly) that such persons are associated with particular systems of belief that would not be congruent with their own beliefs. However, their experience at the FNU was different. They claimed that being heard seemed to allow a deepening and strengthening of their beliefs without their being directed to believe in a particular way, which would have enhanced their suffering.

Unfortunately, at the time of the research interviews, Bill was experiencing a recurrence of leukemia and underwent a bone marrow transplant. Myrna offered her insight during the research interviews that having the opportunity to speak about their faith beliefs made a positive difference in how they were now dealing with their latest health crisis.

> **Myrna:** They (the nurses at the FNU) were prepared to listen to something that doesn't fit into a specific category of formal religion. And that support made a big difference for us and for the kids. We were really thankful for the sessions and we just kept growing spiritually since then. Until the wheels all fell off in May when the leukemia came back. But I think the fact that we were there and we had those sessions helped us to deal with it better this time.

Comments/Reflections

These powerful, reflective comments by Myrna are not only tremendously gratifying to us as a clinical team, but also indicate how changes can continue to reverberate for some time and be useful when further illness challenges or crises occur. As too often happens, this family had not previously met any health professionals who had an interest in their illness and suffering or in their spiritual beliefs about their suffering, even though they had experienced two previous life-threatening situations.

Health professionals missed the privilege of hearing and learning from Bill and Myrna about their current spiritual beliefs.

 Bill and Myrna believed that all experience, including experiences of suffering, occurred for the purpose of learning. It seemed, however, that Bill's suffering was influenced in part because these beliefs were inadequate to address his experience for now. He seemed to hold this belief intellectually, but not in his heart. Myrna, however, found these beliefs to contain much hope for her and she believed that if Bill would simply remember and hold onto this belief, if only he would look for the learning contained in this present experience, his suffering would be eased (McLeod, 2003).

The following is another therapeutic narrative in which Juliet opened space to the spiritual by commenting and reflecting on Bill's previous disclosure that he has reconnected with God since being diagnosed with leukemia. In our practice at the FNU, once family members share that they have a belief in God or a higher power, we inquire if they pray about their condition, and if so, what exactly do they pray? Understanding the nature of the prayer is another path to learning wherein lies the greatest suffering or anguish. Generally, we pray about what we are most troubled about, and this is usually based on the questions that we keep asking ourselves. In Bill's internal conversations with himself, he was continuously asking, "What am I supposed to do... push or not push? What does the future hold for me? What am I supposed to be doing"? We are particularly interested in knowing if a person believes that his prayers are being answered or not and whether this increases or decreases suffering. Notice that Juliet beautifully connected what is most troubling for Bill, his uncertainty about his future, to his praying.

> **JT:** The team was remembering the last session when we were talking about spiritual changes and how you believe that there is a God out there and they were just wondering if you pray about what the future holds for you.

Bill: Yes. I do. But there are no answers. I say "God, please show me the way." And nothing is coming yet. You know, I thank Him for my life. I do not want Him thinking that I do not appreciate because I do, but there's got to be something more. And I am not getting the answer and I do not know whether it's—like you don't expect Him to yell out what the answer is, you know, but I still don't know even if it is job opportunities or even what my direction is. Yeah, I pray to God.

JT: So since God has not kind of thrown out these answers yet, what do you think His answer might be?

Bill: I don't know. 'Cause it's got to be something. Because it is awfully traumatic, what I went through. But maybe it is nothing. Like maybe I am waiting for an answer—maybe there is not an answer. I don't know.

Myrna: But we believe that everything that we go through in our lives good and bad is a learning experience, right?

Bill: Yeah.

Mryna: ...and that there is *something* that we had to learn by going through what you went through—what we went through together. And that—what? (Bill put his head down in his hands.)

Bill: No—go ahead.

Myrna: And that everything good and bad is a learning experience and that you have to learn something from this experience that is going to affect what you are going to do. You did not stick around just to sit at home

Bill: (defensively) I know. I know that.

Myrna: ...and do what you are doing. The path is

there—you just have to be patient for it to come be-cause... .

Bill: It is hard to be patient.

Myrna: He believes that—we believe that in each life-time we are here to learn more and that we learn from all our experiences. And we learn a lot about each other and life through these experiences of ill-ness. But I cannot believe that He (God) left you here just to sit at home and worry about what your future is. There is something there—you do have a future.

Bill: I know.

Myrna: But you have got to get out of what you are in to be able to find it. And I do not know how to get you out.

JT: Well, I was actually wondering when he is—or when Bill is feeling like this—do you feel that you have to kind of cheer him up or? You're the one?

Myrna: Yeah. Yeah, I feel like I have to do something for fear—it is not just for him—it is for me. For fear that I will go there with him. Because he goes into a dark place sometimes and I have been there and I do not want to go there. And I have got to keep myself out of it. I can allow him to be there if that is where he needs to be, but it is hard. It is hard to say, "well he has just got to go through this, you know."

Comments/Reflections

McLeod (2003), in her interpretive inquiry study, understood this piece of clinical dialogue as showing that Bill's "beliefs were proving to be inadequate to address his suffering. Whereas previously such beliefs provided meaning in his life, they brought no comfort in the midst of this suffering." She continued her interpretation by offering the idea that Myrna held the "belief that all of life's experiences were given to us for the purpose of learning something important. If Bill could simply find that learning, he would find purpose in life and his suffering (and Myrna's fear) would be resolved."

Each individual has numerous beliefs operating and emerging every day, about every situation and every person encountered. But not all beliefs matter; not all beliefs invite an emotional or physiological response (Wright et al., 1996). The beliefs that do matter are our core beliefs. We all possess core beliefs, which are personal and often unconscious. Core beliefs are fundamental to how we approach the world; they are the basic concepts by which we live. Our core beliefs are our identity and are accompanied by intense affective and physiological responses. Core beliefs are the "beliefs that matter" within our relationships and within significant events in our lives, such as illness.

Therefore, when differences arise between family members around their core beliefs, particularly in the midst of much suffering and a life-threatening illness, it adds additional suffering and strain even in the best of relationships such as Bill and Myrna's. For example, Bill "no longer found the belief that there was learning in his suffering of any comfort. His struggle to reinterpret this belief provoked strong feelings and fear for Myrna, yet her fear was not that he had no belief that was comforting exactly. Her thought was that *if only* Bill would find spiritual meaning in his current situation, Myrna could let go of some of the fear that she was holding for Bill" (McLeod, 2003). Bringing forth Bill and Myrna's suffering about the illness and its dramatic aftermath through particular and skillful questioning triggered new reflections about the illness and their lives. Myrna had been so fearful that she even worried about suicide with Bill. However, by having a frank discussion about his beliefs and bringing her fears forward, Myrna was now substantially less worried that Bill would end his life through suicide. Of course, the interactional pattern was now shifted! When Myrna was less worried, she was able to allow more suffering talk from Bill. Now there was less need on her part to stifle his expressions of suffering with her spiritual beliefs, but rather could support him even if his beliefs were dramatically different from hers.

 Many of us do not reflect deeply on the religious beliefs, stories, and teachings of our faith traditions until confronted with a question. Often such teachings have a taken-for-grantedness that does not invite questioning. Within a given faith community, however, there is often (if not always) more than one way to understand a given idea, belief, or scripture. One might even argue, that with reflection, no one understands such teachings in *exactly* the same way. New understandings often do evolve in the midst of the questions that we may not yet have confronted, either individually, as a family, or even as a faith community." (McLeod, 2003, p. 178)

This particular case example, I hope, provides the reader with another illustration of the conceptualization and usefulness of the Trinity Model (see Chapter 4). The example also illustrates the application of many of the guideposts highlighted in this chapter.

The clinical work with this courageous and loving family was most rewarding and gratifying. Both Bill and Myrna's suffering was dramatically reduced through many emotional, cognitive, and behavioral changes that occurred during the therapeutic process. They regained their hope for the future and Bill was able to once again find meaning and purpose to his life. Also, powerful healing conversations facilitated by Juliet also occurred between the couple and their sons as preferences for future illness crises were clarified. But this positive and effective clinical work could not have taken place without the reverencing that occurred between Bill and Myrna and Juliet. As their therapeutic relationship unfolded in each session, their profound respect and awe for one another deepened. The evidence for the reverencing in their relationship was the numerous conversations of affirmation and affection that were brought forth in each meeting (Wright et al., 1996). Plus, the clinical team also had a special affection for this family and the family for them!

This family's clinical involvement with the FNU was in 2000. It is with great sadness that I must also tell of the passing of Bill from a recurrence of his leukemia at the end of 2002. We are very grateful and indebted to this family for their generosity of spirit in so willingly giving their permission to share our clinical work with them at the FNU. It is hoped that their story will provide numerous health professionals who read this book with some new ideas for their practice with individuals and families. In so doing, I trust that I have honored Bill's contribution to our learning as a clinical team and the legacy to his family in a manner that is respectful and loving. Of course, the names of these people were changed for reasons of confidentiality, but their spirits that shine through on the pages of this text are not anonymous.

Concluding Thoughts

I offer the clinical guideposts presented in this chapter as practices that might even be thought of as spiritual care practices. Can all nurses offer spiritual care practices in their work with individuals and families? Perhaps not. Perhaps there is some self-selection among nurses who choose to work in pediatric oncology, palliative care, family nursing, long-term care, hospice, or nursing the wounded in times of war or natural disasters. These nurses are quite aware that suffering, dying, and grieving are an integral part of these particular practice areas. I concur with McLeod (2003), who recommends that spiritual care practices must include conversations about beliefs and the meaning of illness in their lives and relationships, conversations about suffering, plus mentoring and life experiences. But even then, some nurses may simply choose, consciously or unconsciously, not to practice in areas where suffering is prominent or front and center. But this is not to judge one health professional as being more valued than another. It is best when we practice where there is the best fit of our competencies, knowledge, and passion. And certainly there is work enough for all.

References

Andersen, T. (1987). The reflecting team: Dialogue and meta-dialogue in clinical work. *Family Process, 26,* 415–428.

Andersen, T. (1991). Basic concepts and practical considerations. In T. Andersen (Ed.), *The reflecting team. Dialogues and dialogues about the dialogues* (pp. 15–41). New York: Norton.

Bateson, G. (1972). *Steps to an ecology of mind.* New York: Ballantine Books.

Cousins, N. (1989). *Beliefs become biology* (videotape). Victoria, British Columbia, Canada: University of Victoria.

Donoghue, P.J., & Siegel, M.E. (1992). *Sick and tired of feeling sick and tired: Living with invisible chronic illness.* New York: Norton.

Dossey, B.M. (2000). *Florence Nightingale: Mystic, visionary, healer.* Springhouse, PA: Springhouse Corporation.

Dossey, L. (1993). *Healing words: The power of prayer and the practice of medicine.* San Francisco: Harper.

Sections of this chapter have been reprinted with permission from Wright, L.M. (1999). Spirituality, suffering, and beliefs: The soul of healing with families. In Walsh, F. (Ed.), *Spiritual Resources in Family Therapy.* New York: Guilford.

Frank, A.W. (1994). Interrupted stories, interrupted lives. *Second Opinion, 20*(1), 11–18.

Frank, A.W. (1995). *The wounded storyteller: Body, illness, and ethics.* Chicago: The University of Chicago Press.

Kleinman, D. (1988). *The illness narrative.* New York: Basic Books.

Levac, A.M., McLean, S., Wright, L.M., Bell, J.M., Ann, & Fred (1998). A Reader's Theatre intervention to managing grief: Post-therapy reflections by a family and a clinical team. *Journal of Marital and Family Therapy, 24*(1), 81–94.

Maturana, H.R. (1998). Reality: The search for objectivity or the quest for a compelling argument. *Irish Journal of Psychology, 9*(1), 25–83.

Maturana, H.R., & Varela, F.G. (1992). *The tree of knowledge: The biological roots of human understanding* (rev. ed.). Boston, MA: Shambhala.

McLeod, D.L. (2003). Opening space for the spiritual: Therapeutic conversations with families living with serious illness. Unpublished doctoral dissertation, University of Calgary, Alberta, Canada.

McNeil, J.A. (1998). Coping: Pain questionnaire to hospitalized patients. *Journal of Pain and Symptom Management, 16*(1), 29–40.

Remen, R.N. (1993). Wholeness. In B. Moyers (Ed.), *Healing and the mind* (pp. 343–363). New York: Doubleday.

Thomas, G. (January 6, 1997). Doctors who pray: How the medical community is discovering the healing power of prayer. *Christianity Today,* pp. 20–28.

Wright, L.M. (1989). When clients ask questions: Enriching the therapeutic conversation. *The Family Therapy Networker, 13*(6), 15–16.

Wright, L.M., & Levac, A.M. (1992). The non-existence of non-compliant families: The influence of Humberto Maturana. *Journal of Advanced Nursing,* 17, 913–917.

Wright, L.M., Bell, J.M., Watson, W.L., & Tapp, D. (1995). The influence of the beliefs of nurses: A clinical example of a post-myocardial-infarction couple. *Journal of Family Nursing, 1*(3), 238–256.

Wright, L.M., Watson, W.L., & Bell, J.M. (1996). *Beliefs: The heart of healing in families and illness.* New York: Basic Books.

6

Connecting the Personal and the Professional in Matters of Suffering, Spirituality, and Illness

Suffering and joy teach us, if we allow them, how to make the leap of empathy, which transports us into the soul and heart of another person. In those transparent moments we know other people's joys and sorrows, and we care about their concerns as if they were our own.

Fritz Williams

Important ingredients that we need to put in place are the ability and maturity to integrate our personal and professional lives in matters of suffering and spirituality. This is imperative to bring forth more genuine therapeutic conversations with patients and families. Of course, there will be differences in our ability as a result of age and life experiences. Some nurses and other health professionals are young in years; others may be inexperienced in matters of suffering; or perhaps their spiritual beliefs are different from, or less well developed than, those of their patients. Even if there are some shortcomings in life experience or in health professionals' own spiritual development, they can still be enormously helpful to patients and their families in their encounters with suffering. Nurses and other health professionals can be compassionate and caring if they embrace a particular way of being with patients (e.g., engaging in spiritual practices such as those outlined in Chapter 5); if they have a model for practice, such as the Trinity Model, to inform and guide their practice about suffering and spirituality in the context of illness (see Chapter 4); and if they have some clinical guideposts to mark the way in their practice (see Chapter 5). All of these suggestions and ideas will add to our own learning of how to be vigilant and cognizant about the reciprocity between our personal and professional lives in regard to suffering and spirituality.

Personal to Professional

How do we connect our personal experiences to our professional lives in ways that can bring forth greater compassion and understanding for those who suffer and are in our care? One such experience helped me to know more profoundly what I call the phenomenon of "living in a different world" experience of those who live daily with serious illness, disability, or loss.

I wrote the following in my journal during the final few months of my mother's life:

> Dad is away at the cottage for a few days for some much needed respite. I am staying overnight with Mom. It was a very tiring evening again, as my mom is not eating and in lots of pain. I was so glad to be here when the doctor arrived. He is going to titrate her meds up again. Incredible how these pain meds can go up and up. Despite all this, we did have some pleasant moments and of course Mom and I have different kinds of conversations when Dad is not present. But it continues to be very difficult for me to observe my mother so ill and in so much pain. Watching the deterioration inch by inch of her body and life is for me mile by mile suffering!!

Indeed, during this time of "mile by mile" suffering, I was much more acutely aware and in tune with the suffering of others, particularly with one friend who was dying at the same time as my mother, and another who was encountering a serious illness, in addition to the families with whom I was working at the Family Nursing

Unit at the University of Calgary. I found I had a greater compassion, a greater kinship, and a greater understanding for the sufferings of others, whether they were friends or patients.

Surprisingly to me, I did not experience being surrounded by suffering both personally and professionally as particularly onerous; rather, it was comforting to be in the presence of others whose lives were also engulfed in suffering. There seemed to be an unspoken bond among those of us who were suffering simply in the way we were experiencing our world. My suffering seemed even to be enhanced and difficult in the presence of others whom I judged, unfairly I admit, as being too frivolous, too superficial, too concerned with life's trivia, or even too happy. But they were simply living their lives, experiencing joy, as we all do when suffering has not caught our attention for a time or, worse yet, consumed us. Yes, those who suffer do live in a different world from those who are living their fortunate lives without deep suffering!

Professional to Personal

Frequently we do not recognize or give credit to the numerous times when our caring for patients and families brings great benefits to our personal lives and relationships. We can be under the illusion that we are doing all the "giving" and, we hope, healing by diminishing or reducing suffering in our caring for patients. We may not recognize that the stories of suffering, strength, compassion, endurance, and love that we hear and witness in the midst of serious illness are offering us hope, inspiration, and even guidance for our own lives. Nursing is certainly not a one-way street of offerings where we give our best professional knowledge, opinions, and treatment; rather, the patients and families with whom we meet are also changing and benefiting our lives, perhaps more than we are aware of or care to acknowledge.

One such example for me was a young man who was diagnosed with multiple sclerosis (MS). When I met him, he was just in his early 30s and was experiencing great emotional suffering from his condition. During my meeting with him and his parents, I inquired, "What's the toughest part about managing MS every day and coping with it?" This therapeutic conversation was not about symptoms, medication, or treatment, but rather about this young man's illness experience; the specific intention was to understand the potential or actual areas of suffering. He gave a poignant response: "Things that seemed so trivial I can't really do any more. They're not really important things, but everyone does them."

This young man helped me to learn and to remember that many of the daily tasks and routines that are normally out of our awareness and taken for granted are gone out of his capabilities and into his awareness in the context of illness. I was reminded of my experience in assisting my mother with bathing, dressing, and eating. Turning on the water taps, fastening your own brassiere, and spreading jam on your toast are

just a few of the things that, as this young man
taught me, are "not really important things, but
everyone does them." That is, everyone does
them except this young man, my mother when
living, and countless others for whom these
tasks and routines accentuate their dependence
on and difference from others (Wright, Watson,
& Bell, 1996). Serious illness often disrupts
taken-for-granted ways of being in the world.
Such disruptions often lead to suffering and
therefore can trigger a search for meaning. This
one example of my own learning I have often
passed on and transferred to other patients and
families with whom I have worked. I now fully appreciate that the inability to perform everyday
tasks produces constant and unrelenting "pin-
prick" reminders to those who have a serious illness or disability that their lives have
substantially, and often irreversibly, changed.
This is simply one example of the great learning
that I have gained from patients and families
with whom I have worked. My best learning experiences always come from the patients themselves, supplemented by the professional
literature and my own and others' research.

Our Life Experience Is Not Our Patients' Life Experience

Often there is a tendency and temptation among
health-care providers to offer their own understandings, their own "better" meanings or beliefs

for clients' suffering experiences with serious illness. For example, one family related to me that after their son's death from a motor vehicle accident, a nurse suggested, "It must be your son's time; otherwise he would not have died so young." But these supposedly well-meaning comments were not comforting to this family. It did not decrease their suffering. As the family related, "Maybe that was this nurse's explanation or understanding, but it was not ours. We are still searching for a satisfying explanation for our son's death." One way to avoid this trap of prematurely offering explanations or advice to reduce suffering is to remain insatiably curious about how clients and their families are managing in the midst of suffering, especially what they believe and what meaning they give to their suffering (Wright et al., 1996).

Being insatiably curious can be one of the most rewarding, enlightening, and educating experiences for nurses, both personally and professionally. How do those who suffer with serious illness make sense of their lives? How are their family members responding and reacting? What have they found that helps them to cope? What influence, if any, do their spiritual or religious beliefs have on their suffering?

Health professionals who are insatiably curious put on the armor of prevention against blame, judgment, or the need to be "right." Asking therapeutic or reflexive questions (Tomm, 1987; Wright & Leahey, 2000; Wright et al., 1996) invites people to explore and reflect on the meanings that they derive from their suffering, not those of the nurse. In the reflections in the therapeutic conversations we have with our patients, we hope that healing will be triggered as new thoughts, ideas, or solutions come forth and are pondered, and as patients consider how best to live their lives with illness.

Reflections are invited through very deliberate and thoughtful questions. Examples of questions that I have found very useful to invite curiosity are the following:

- ❀ What questions do you find yourself asking these days (about your illness or your suffering)?
- ❀ Have you come to any understanding about your suffering?
- ❀ How do you make sense of your suffering?
- ❀ What parts of your suffering are hardest to make sense of? What's that like for you?
- ❀ Does your story or explanation of suffering match the stories of those who matter most to you?
- ❀ How are these stories the same or different from those offered by health professionals?
- ❀ Does suffering seem to assign words or stories to your personality?

Of course, we also learn from families for future clinical work and our own relationships. Therefore there are questions we need to pose to ourselves about the influence of our clinical work. It is our routine practice as a clinical team in the FNU to ask ourselves the following questions:

❋ What will I take away or have learned from this family that will benefit me in future work with other families?

❋ What will I take away or have learned that will help me in my personal life?

❋ What will I never forget about this family?

❋ What belief(s) of mine was (were) challenged or confirmed through my clinical work with this individual or family?

Sometimes sufferers seek understanding in words, images, and metaphors that have the potential to provide relief. One young man with whom I worked experienced severe back pain after a serious cycling accident. He offered the idea that when his physical suffering from back pain was at its worst, he found some relief when he imagined himself on a beach listening to the sound of the waves. Conversely, he found that his back pain was enhanced when he and his wife had a conflict.

In my life and in the lives of those for whom I have cared, it has been my experience that, after time, some of the stories and meanings of suffering lose their usefulness and there is a need for new conversations that yield fresh meanings, that "renarratize" or bring hope.

After one particularly difficult visit with my mother, I found myself unable to watch or participate when her emaciated, quadriplegic body was turned one more time by her lovely and compassionate caregivers. As I walked down the hallway from her room, feeling the salty tears on my cheeks, I became aware of a conversation that I was having with myself. "What more can I learn from Mom's suffering? I have nothing more to learn. I cannot watch this suffering of my mother nor understand it any more." The previous stories of why my mother suffered, of why my family and I suffered, and of what might be learned from it, which had been so useful in the past, had now worn thin! I needed a new story, a new meaning, and a new ray of hope. When "meaning making" breaks down, our explanatory conversations and their particular meanings lose their vitality, and we often find that suffering, conflict, or alienation is not far behind.

So what does help in these moments? I have found the words of a rabbi written around 930 AD to be most profound and consistent with my own beliefs. He said, "Comfort the sufferer by the promise of healing, even when you are not confident, for thus you may assist his natural powers" (Israeli, Manhig HaRofiem). Yes, as health professionals we need to offer the promise of healing and hope to the very end! We need to assist our patients in finding the kind of hope that is meaningful for them. Of course, this does not necessarily mean the kind of hope that someone will be cured of illness or their loss reversed, but rather the hope that they will find meaning in their suffering, that they will know that their life is still important to the lives of others and, most important, to themselves, despite the changes their illness has brought to their lives and to their most intimate relationships.

Learning and Offering through Therapeutic Letters

Another way to connect the personal and professional in matters of suffering and spirituality is through the use of therapeutic letters. Therapeutic letters have been used at the FNU for some 17 years. Although for some time many clinicians have written therapeutic letters to clients to invite family members to sessions, offer ideas and suggestions, summarize therapeutic work, or solidify change, it was White and Epston's (1990) creative book *Narrative Means to Therapeutic Ends* that catapulted letter writing into the therapeutic mainstream. In our efforts to write therapeutic letters (Wright et al., 1996), we have found them to be a marvelous medium for carrying into homes, minds, hearts, and spirits of family members, in sealed personally addressed envelopes, such things as:

* Commendations highlighting individual and family members' strengths, resources, and competencies
* Questions we would have or could have asked in a session
* Words, phrases, and ideas that particularly stood out for us from a session
* Highlights of our work with a family and what we learned from our work with them
* Any therapeutic and professional advice, suggestions, and opinions

At the end of our clinical work with a family, we routinely send a letter that is a long conversation of affirmation and affection (Wright et al., 1996) consisting of two major components: what we have learned from the family and what we believed we offered the family in the form of our professional suggestions, ideas, and advice. Below is an example of such a therapeutic letter that illustrates the professional and personal learning from this family plus what we believed we offered the family. This was the closing letter sent from our clinical team to the family discussed in Chapter 5.

 Dear Bill and Myrna,

Greetings from the Family Nursing Unit! As part of completing our clinical work with families, we send a closing letter as a summary and record of our time spent together. We met on five different occasions. On three of these occasions, we had the opportunity to work with you as a couple, and on two other occasions, your sons were able to join us as well.

We would like to share what we learned from your family and what we believe we offered you in these sessions. Your presenting request, Bill, was for advice on how to cope with your sense of not being a whole person as a result of the experiences you had after your stroke. Myrna, your presenting request was for advice about whether you should be pushing Bill to accept his losses and new limits and just "let him be" in this space of deep grief, or whether you should be pushing him to fight back and define his own limits. Even though it has been over a month since the last time we were in contact with you, due to the winter holidays, we are still deeply moved and thankful for the opportunity to work with your family.

What We Learned from Your Family

1. We learned about how love between a courageous husband and wife, and two amazing sons, cannot be diminished even in the face of illness. We further learned that the love between family members can grow, strengthen, and evolve as a result of hardships in life. This love can be expressed and experimented with in a variety of new ways so that communication between one another can flourish.

2. Bill, you taught us what pushing the limits really means. Through pushing the limits you have taught us that it is possible to gain control over illnesses that at first can have a grip on your sense of self. We learned from you that making a contribution to the world is what living is truly about. As a result of your motivation, you have made many contributions to your family and to society in general. You have contributed to our own learning at the Family Nursing Unit by showing us what courage and love for a spouse and children can accomplish.

3. Myrna, we have learned from you about unconditional love. Unconditional, fearless love for your husband and your sons is what you demonstrated to us. You taught us that as a loving wife, and as a loving mother, you wanted to protect your family from feeling

the wrath of the illness. You have taught us what strength a woman, wife, and mother can have, and the significant influence she can have over family illness experiences.

What We Believe We Offered You

1. We offered Bill the idea of pushing the limits, and finding his own limits as a result of the stroke. We suggested to you not to give up and not allow the illness to have control over your sense of self. We offered Myrna, wife and the caregiver, the idea of not pushing the limits. We offered you the idea, Myrna, to take more breaks from caregiving, but not of course from loving.

2. We offered you the idea of going to the "sex shop." We suggested that perhaps a way you could push the limits was to experiment in your sexual relations. We invited you to go and explore the sex shop, and explore with each other in order that you would be able to continue to find physical pleasure from each other. We offered you the idea of not letting the illness have the upper hand in terms of your intimate relationship, and to push the limits around your sexuality.

3. We offered you the idea to "speak the unspeakable." We invited you to speak about things that perhaps you wanted to speak about but did not know how to approach the conversation or were afraid to approach the conversation. We offered you the idea that healing arises out of speaking the unspeakable, and by the end of our time together

you were demonstrating to us how to speak the unspeakable, and you were finding healing from within. We were also impressed with your sons, who were also able to "speak the unspeakable" and thus have an opportunity to put some of their illness experiences in their place.

In closing, we would like to remind you that you will be contacted in about six months' time to be invited to participate in a follow-up study, intended to improve our clinical practice with families. We would also like to offer you a final Shakespearean thought:

To be or not to be, that is the question,
Whether 'tis nobler in the mind to suffer
The slings and arrows of outrageous fortune
Or to take arms against a sea of troubles,
And, by opposing, end them.

William Shakespeare: *Hamlet*

Warmest regards,
Juliet Thornton, BScN, RN
Masters Student
Lorraine M. Wright, RN, PhD
Director of the Family Nursing Unit
Professor, Faculty of Nursing
And other members of the clinical team

We have received incredibly positive feedback about the healing aspects of these letters that we write to families. And this family was no different. They reported 6 months later to our research assistant that they found this letter very helpful and hopeful in their healing process. To understand more about the effect and usefulness of these letters to individuals and families,

Moules (2000a, 2000b; 2002) conducted a most comprehensive and eloquent piece of qualitative research in the FNU that was the first of its kind regarding therapeutic letters between nurses and families. It appears from this research that therapeutic letters serve as a particularly effective healing balm for suffering and can be reapplied when suffering re-emerges. Families report that they often go back to these letters and reread them when they feel the need. Letter writing also provides an opportunity for clinicians to reflect and then offer the family another perspective on their suffering that might bring forth hope. I believe these letters serve as inspiration and express admiration for how the human spirit deals with adversity and suffering for both client and clinician.

Learning and Offering through Commendations

Another aspect of therapeutic letters and therapeutic conversations is the opportunity to offer commendations (Bohn , Wright, & Moules, 2003; Houger Limacher, 2003; Houger Limacher & Wright, 2003; Wright & Leahey, 2000; and Wright et al., 1996). Commendations tend to highlight individual and family members' strengths, competencies, and resources. In another fluent and moving piece of research conducted by Houger Limacher (2003), she focused on the intervention of commendations as offered in the clinical practice at the FNU. A key discov-

ery was that both families and nurses reported
and reiterated the value and power of commendations that brought forth "goodness" and
helped alleviate their suffering (Houger Limacher,
2003). This bringing forth of "goodness" becomes a relational phenomenon in the context
of the nurse/patient/family relationship. Commendations have the power to create and bring
forth "goodness," or what I refer to as "particular kinds of persons" who possess a "particular
way of being in the world." This particular kind
of person and way of being in clinical practice
are represented by a person who looks for
strengths amid suffering, hope amid despair, and
meaning amid confusion. "We become our conversations and we generate the conversations
that we become" (Maturana & Varela, 1992).
These types of therapeutic conversations entered
into by health providers who bring forth "goodness" are what I believe form the structure and
foundation of spiritual practices. This way of
being in the world connects and integrates our
personal lives to our professional lives, and vice
versa.

Hope for the Future

There is hope for the future in incorporating spiritual care practices by connecting our personal
and professional selves in matters of suffering
and spirituality. This hope lies, of course, in the
young, enthusiastic, and caring graduate and un-
dergraduate nursing students whom we are privileged to know. I have full confidence in their

abilities as I hear and observe their growth in knowledge, skill in therapeutic conversations, and compassion in working with those who suffer.

One such outstanding student was Shari Laliberte. I received this inspiring, reflective, and precious e-mail from her when she received her Master's in Nursing degree specializing in family systems nursing. "I just want to thank you from the bottom of my heart again for everything. And after more thought, the one thing I take with me from my studies, I was reminded of the night I watched the movie 'My Life as a House' and how I almost emailed you. What I was going to mention is my deep gratitude for how you have re-minded me/reconnected me to our shared humanity and spirituality in this work...and how you have given life to these core sacred ways of being with families. This is the primary gift that I take with me and which I hope to share with others!" And this email from Shari was, of course, my gift!

Spirit Matters

When we reduce or diminish suffering, be it through our therapeutic conversations or thera-peutic letters, we are touching or reawakening dampened, discouraged, and distraught spirits. Illness, and often the suffering experiences that accompany illness, can demoralize and oppress lives, relationships, and our very spirits. Lerner (2000) says it so succinctly in the title of his book, *Spirit Matters*. I believe the more that we are able to connect suffering and spirituality in our professional and personal lives, the more we as individuals will be well integrated and well equipped to succor and support those who suffer. Yes, spirit matters.

References

Bohn, U., Wright, L.M., & Moules, N.J. (2003). A family systems nursing interview following a myocardial infarction: The power of commendations. *Journal of Family Nursing, 9*(2), 151–165.

Houger Limacher, L., & Wright, L.M. (2003). Commendations: Listening to the silent side of a family intervention. *Journal of Family Nursing, 9*(2), 130–135.

Houger Limacher, L. (2003). Commendations: The healing potential of one family systems nursing intervention. Unpublished doctoral thesis: University of Calgary.

Lerner, M. (2000). *Spirit matters*. Charlottesville, VA: Walsch Books, an imprint of Hampton Roads Publishing Co.

Maturana, H.R., & Varela, F.G. (1992). *The tree of knowledge: The biological roots of human understanding* (rev. ed.). Boston, MA: Shambhala.

Moules, N.J. (2000a). Nursing on paper: The art and mystery of therapeutic letters in clinical work with families experiencing illness. Doctoral thesis: University of Calgary.

Moules, N.J. (2002b). Therapy on paper: Therapeutic letters and the tone of relationship. *Journal of Systemic Therapies, 22*(1), 33–49.

Moules, N.J. (2002). Nursing on paper: Therapeutic letters in nursing practice. *Nursing Inquiry, 9*(2), 104–113.

Tomm, K. (1987). Interventive interviewing: Part II. Reflexive questioning as a means to enable self-healing. *Family Process, 26*(6), 167–183.

White, M., & Epston, D. (1990). *Narrative means to therapeutic ends.* New York: W.W. Norton.

Wright, L.M., & Leahey, M. (2000), 3rd ed. *Nurses and families: A guide to family assessment and intervention.* Philadelphia: FA Davis Co.

Wright, L.M., Watson, W.L., & Bell, J.M. (1996). *Beliefs: The heart of healing in families and illness.* New York: Basic Books.

Epilogue

How does one end a book on spirituality, suffering, and illness? When I reread what I have written, I know that this has been the most "personal" academic book that I have ever authored! But I suppose that, in matters of spirit and suffering, how can it be otherwise? Perhaps this text really is **only** personal, with some academic sprinklings.

However this book may be described or named, my sincere hope is that within its pages we have all been invited and called, myself included, to further reflections about suffering, spirituality, and illness and have reaffirmed what we are doing that is useful in our professional lives and practice. I hope that the reader has gleaned some new understanding and ideas for listening, caring for, and inviting conversations about suffering and spirituality with patients and their families so that opportunities for healing may begin. It is hoped that the Trinity Model (see Chapter 4) and the Clinical Guideposts (see Chapter 5) will be very specific and new additions to health professionals' practice. And, of course, that all of the knowledge and healing will occur within and between the relationships of the "trinity" of patient, family, and health-care providers.

Under the blows of mortal experience, those who suffer from serious illness, loss, or disability need comfort, hope, and, above all, the knowledge and reassurance that they are still cherished. This kind of practice is indeed spiritual and one that offers a great opportunity and blessing for all health professionals.

Index

Note: Page numbers followed by f indicate figures.

Acknowledgment of suffering, 149–151
Affiliation (church affiliation). *See also* Religion.
  and assumed synonymity of religion with
    spirituality, 72
  correlated with health outcomes, 79
Afterlife, judgment in, and fear accompanying
  suffering, 135
Alleviation of suffering, 40. *See also* Healing.
  as focus of nursing, 36. *See also* Nursing.
Answer-seeking, by patient, 18, 155, 164
    questions exemplifying, 16, 45
Appeal, of illness narratives or stories of suffering,
  130
Attendance, at church. *See* Affiliation; Religion.
Attention to suffering, lack of, 36
    reasons for, 46

Bad vs. good Karma, 22
Beliefs, 40, 76, 186
  about illness, 53–54, 113–116
  constraining, 115, 155
  core, 186
  facilitating, 115, 126
    questions introducing, 136–137

Beliefs (*Continued*)
    family systems of, 76
    suffering and spirituality in relation to, 112f
    Trinity Model encompassing, 112f, 113–128
Buddhist view, of suffering, 22–23

Care, spiritual, 73, 84–87, 89, 93
    nursing responsibility for, 67
    validation and, for soul, 77
"Cheer-up" interference, with illness narratives, 165, 169
Chemotherapy recipients, husbands of, suffering by, 52
Church affiliation. *See also* Religion.
    and assumed synonymity of religion with spirituality, 72
    and attendance, correlated with health outcomes, 79
Closing letter, in epistolary therapy, 204
    example of, covering knowledge gained from family, 205–206
      covering knowledge provided to family, 206–207
Commendations, and healing, 56, 208–209
Constraining beliefs, 115, 155
Conversations, therapeutic, 44, 56, 147–190
    environment for, 55
    inviting-of-reflections gambit in, 173
      change effected via, 177
      suffering made understood via, 158, 159, 178, 200
      team approach to, 173
    "meaning-centered," 32
Core beliefs, 186

Demoralizing effects, of illness and suffering, 211
Despair, spirituality as protection against, 132
Detachment, from suffering, problems with, 53
Distress, spiritual, 131
    NANDA criteria for, 83
Doctor, praying for patient by, 162

Emotional healing, vs. physical healing, 157
Empathy, in relation to sympathy espoused by
    Florence Nightingale, 65
Emptiness, sufferer's experience of, 43
Enduring, suffering and, 49
Epistolary therapy, 56, 203–208
    closing letter in, 204
        example of, covering knowledge gained from
            family, 205–206
            covering knowledge provided to family,
            206–207
    reapplicability of, 208
Everyday life. *See also* Experience.
    stories of suffering and spirituality in, 2, 6–29.
        See also Suffering, stories of.
        import of, 30–32
Experience. *See also* Everyday life.
    personal, in relation to professional life, 195–198
        vs. patient's life experience, 198–202

Facilitating beliefs, 115, 126
    questions introducing, 136–137
Family (families), 75
    belief systems of, 76
    coverage of knowledge provided by or to, in
        sample closing therapeutic letter, 205–207
    response of, to illness, 96

Family (families) (*Continued*)
  spirituality of, 75–77
    individual-spirituality model favored over, 64
  suffering by, 48–51
    emotions exemplifying, among husbands of
      chemotherapy recipients, 52
    intervention research concerning, 51, 52
Family Nursing Unit (University of Calgary), 55
  therapeutic sessions in, 56
    follow-up on, transcript of, 180–181
    opportunities afforded by, necessity of, 57
    team approach to, 173–177
    transcripts of, 117–127, 166–167, 170–172,
      183–185
Fear, as component of suffering, 43
  judgment in afterlife and, 135
FNU. *See* Family Nursing Unit (University of Calgary).
Fretting, as component of suffering, 43

Good vs. bad Karma, 22
Goodness, commendations eliciting, 209

Harmonious interconnectedness, and spirituality,
  69
Healing, 128, 156
  commendations and, 56, 208–209
  emotional vs. physical, 157
  epistolary cure and, 203–208. *See also* Letters,
    therapeutic.
  nurse's role in, as witness to stories of suffering,
    37
  physical vs. emotional, 157
  promise of, importance of, 202
  "talking cure" and, 147–190. *See also*
    Conversations, therapeutic.

Health outcomes, religion and, 79
    spirituality and, 81
Health-care environment, pervasiveness of suffering
    in, 36
Holistic nursing, 67
Hope, nursing students as source of, 210

Illness, 38. *See also* Illness narrative(s).
    beliefs about, 53–54, 113–116
    changes wrought by, recognition of, 197, 198
    demoralizing effects of, 211
    families' experience of, 96
    questioning patient about effects of, 38–39, 197
    suffering due to. *See* Suffering.
    twentieth-century perceptions of, 65
Illness Beliefs Model, 53–54
Illness narrative(s), 37, 38, 44, 157. *See also*
        Suffering, stories of.
    appeal of, 130
    interference with, by listener's "cheering-up"
        attempts, 165, 169
    inviting-listening-witnessing approach to, 77
    vs. medical narrative, 37
Illness stories. *See* Illness narrative(s).
Inattention, to suffering, 36
    causes of, 46
Individual spirituality, 64
    conceptual models focusing on, to exclusion of
        family spirituality, 64
Inner strengths, and spirituality, 69
Inner vs. outer talk, 181
Interconnectedness, and spirituality, 69
Intervention research, family suffering as subject
        of, 51, 52
    spirituality as subject of, 93

Inviting-listening-witnessing approach, to stories of
       illness, 77
   to stories of suffering, 37–38, 151–155, 158
Inviting-of-reflections gambit, in therapeutic conver-
       sations, 173
       change effected via, 177
       suffering made understood via, 158, 159, 178,
           200
       team approach to, 173

Job, as personification of suffering, 153
Judgment, in afterlife, and fear accompanying suf-
       fering, 135

Karma, good vs. bad, 22

Language of religion vs. spirituality, 90–91
Learning, from research. *See* Research.
Letters, therapeutic, 56, 203–208
       re-reading of, 208
       summary components of, 204
           example of, covering knowledge gained from
               family, 205–206
               covering knowledge provided to family,
                   206–207
Life experiences. *See also* Everyday life.
   nurses' vs. patients', 198–202
   professional lives in relation to, 195–198
Listening, to stories of suffering, 151–155
Love, and reverencing, 161

"Meaning-centered" therapeutic conversations, 32.
       See also Therapeutic conversations.
Medical narrative, 37
   vs. illness narrative, 37. *See also* Illness narra-
       tive(s).

Medical perspective, on suffering, 45
Mystery, unfolding, and spirituality, 69

NANDA (North American Nursing Diagnosis
  Association) criteria, for spiritual distress, 83
Needs, spiritual, 82, 83, 91
Nightingale, Florence, on spiritual focus of
  nursing, 65
  on sympathy, 65
  youth of, dedication beginning in, 148
North American Nursing Diagnosis Association
  (NANDA) criteria, for spiritual distress, 83
Nurse(s). *See also* Nursing.
  as witness to stories of suffering, 37
  connecting personal and professional lives of,
    195–198
  life experience of, vs. patient's life experience,
    198–202
  specialist, self-selection among, 189
  student, as source of hope, 210
Nursing. *See also* Nurse(s).
  family interventions in, 51–52
  history of, institutional religion in, 65
  holistic, 67
  research conducted as part of. *See* Research.
  responsibility for spiritual care in, 67
  spirituality in, 64–68
    Florence Nightingale on, 65
  spirituality-suffering-belief model applied to. *See*
    Trinity model, for nursing.
  suffering as focus of, 36. *See also* Suffering.

Objectification, of spirituality, 91–95
Outer vs. inner talk, 181

Pain, suffering due to, 44

Patient(s). *See also* Family (families).
  answer-seeking by, 18, 155, 164
    questions exemplifying, 16, 45
  as source of information about effects of illness,
    38–39, 197
  introducing facilitating beliefs to, 136–137
  inviting reflections from, to effect change, 177
    to make suffering understood, 158, 159, 178,
      200
  life experience of, vs. nurse's life experience,
    198–202
  praying by, 162
  praying for, by physician, 162
  spiritual preferences of, 88
  suicidal potential of, search for, 121
"Pedagogy of suffering," 39, 143
Personal experience. *See also* Everyday life.
  in relation to professional life, 195–198
  vs. patient's life experience, 198–202
Personal/spiritual dimensions, 68–69
Physical healing, vs. emotional healing, 157
Physician, praying for patient by, 162
Prayer, 162–163, 183
Professional literature. *See* Research.

Questioning of patient, about answer-seeking, 155,
  164
  about effects of illness, 38–39, 197
  about suicidal thoughts, 121
  to introduce facilitating beliefs, 136–137
  to invite reflections on making suffering under-
    stood, 178, 200

Reapplicability, of epistolary therapy, 208
Reflection, soliciting of. *See* Therapeutic conversations, inviting-of-reflections gambit in.

Religion, 4–5, 74
  definition of, 4–5
  health outcomes correlated with, 79
  institutional, in history of nursing, 65
  redemptive prospects in, applied to suffering, 46
  vs. spirituality, 69, 73, 74, 90–91
    persons ignoring dichotomy of, 72, 73
Research, nursing intervention, 51, 52, 93
  proposed subjects of, 54–55
  religion and health as subject of, 79
  spirituality as subject of, 66, 77–78, 80–90, 93
  suffering as subject of, 39, 49, 50, 51, 52, 58
Reverencing, 141, 142, 160, 161, 188
Rumination, as component of suffering, 43

Sadness, vs. sorrow, 42
Self, 77
Self-selection, among nurse-specialists, 189
Sorrow, as component of suffering, 42
  vs. sadness, 42
Soul, 77
  cross-cultural characterizations of, 71–72
Soul care, 77
Specialist nurses, self-selection among, 189
Spirit, 8, 68, 71. *See also* Spirituality.
Spiritual care, 73, 84–87, 89, 93
  nursing responsibility for, 67
Spiritual distress, 131
  NANDA criteria for, 83
Spiritual needs, 82, 83, 91
Spiritual preferences, 88
Spirituality, 4, 69–71
  beliefs and suffering in relation to, 112f
  definitions of, 4, 69–71
  family, 75–77
    individual-spirituality model favored over, 64

Spirituality (*Continued*)
  harmonious interconnectedness and, 69
  health outcomes correlated with, 81
  individual, 64
    conceptual models focusing on, to exclusion of
      family spirituality, 64
  inner strengths and, 69
  nursing in terms of, 64–68
    Florence Nightingale on, 65
  nursing research concerning, 78, 80–90
  objectification of, 91–95
  protection afforded by, against despair, 132
  research concerning, 66, 77–78, 80–90, 93
  suffering and beliefs in relation to, 112f
  suffering in everyday life and, stories of, 2, 6–29.
    See also Suffering, stories of.
      import of, 30–32
  theorizing applied to, 64
    incompleteness of, with regard to family, 64
  Trinity Model encompassing, 112f, 130–142
  unfolding mystery and, 69
  vs. religion, 69, 73, 74, 90–91
    persons ignoring dichotomy of, 72, 73
Spiritual/personal dimensions, 68–69
Strengths, inner, and spirituality, 69
Student nurses, as source of hope, 210
SUFFER mnemonic, 42–43
Suffering, 3, 37, 41, 128–129
  acknowledgment of, 149–151
  alleviation of, 40. *See also* Healing.
    as focus of nursing, 36. *See also* Nursing.
  beliefs and spirituality in relation to, 112f
  Buddhist view of, 22–23
  definitions of, 3, 37, 41, 128–129

demoralizing effects of, 211
detachment from, problems with, 53
educative value claimed for, dismissal of, 45
emptiness characterizing, 43
enduring in relation to, 49
families' experience of, 48–51
  emotions exemplifying, among husbands of
    chemotherapy recipients, 52
  intervention research concerning, 51, 52
fear accompanying, 43
  judgment in afterlife and, 135
fretting occasioned by, 43
illness and. *See* Illness; Illness narrative(s).
inattention to, 36
  causes of, 46
Job as personification of, 153
medical perspective on, 45
multifaceted nature of, 31
  mnemonic for, 42–43
need for alleviating, 40. *See also* Healing.
  as focus of nursing, 36. *See also* Nursing.
pain and, 44
"pedagogy" of, 39, 143
pervasiveness of, in health-care environment, 36
research concerning, 39, 49, 50, 51, 52, 58
rumination as component of, 43
sentiments trivializing, 47, 48, 155, 156
shared, comfort from, 195–196
sorrow as component of, 42
spirituality and beliefs in relation to, 112f
stories of, 157. *See also* Illness narrative(s).
  appeal of, 130
  everyday, 2, 6–29
    import of, 30–32

Suffering (*Continued*)
    finite usefulness of, 201
    inviting-listening-witnessing approach to, 37–38,
      151–155, 158
   temporizing as untoward approach to, 47, 48,
     155, 156
   theological perspectives on, 46
   Trinity Model encompassing, 112f, 128–130
   unfairness perceived in relation to, 42–43
Suicidal thoughts, questioning of patient about,
   121
Sympathy, Florence Nightingale's perception of, 65

Talk, inner vs. outer, 181
"Talking cure." *See* Therapeutic conversations.
Team approach, to FNU therapeutic sessions,
   173–177
Temporizing, as untoward approach to suffering,
   47, 48, 155, 156
Theological perspectives. *See* Religion.
Therapeutic conversations, 44, 56, 147–190
  environment for, 55
  inviting-of-reflections gambit in, 173
    change effected via, 177
    suffering made understood via, 158, 159, 178,
     200
    team approach to, 173
  "meaning-centered," 32
Therapeutic letters, 56, 203–208
  re-reading of, 208
  summary components of, 204
    example of, covering knowledge gained from
      family, 205–206
     covering knowledge provided to family,
      206–207

Trinity Model, for nursing, 110–112, 112f
    belief component of, 113–128
        in relation to suffering and spirituality, 112f
    spirituality component of, 130–142
    in relation to beliefs and suffering, 112f
    suffering component of, 128–130
        in relation to beliefs and spirituality, 112f
    theories/views informing, 110–111
    zone of intersections in, 112, 112f

Unfairness, perception of, as component of suffering, 42–43
Unfolding mystery, and spirituality, 69
University of Calgary Family Nursing Unit, 55
    therapeutic sessions in, 56
        follow-up on, transcript of, 180–181
        opportunities afforded by, necessity of, 57
        team approach to, 173–177
        transcripts of, 117–127, 166–167, 170–172,
            183–185
Unspeakable subjects, broaching of, 119, 206–207

Witnessing, of stories of suffering, 37–38, 151–155,
    158

Zone of intersections, in Trinity Model, 112, 112f